Start Your Own Homemade

Organic Cosmetics Brand

110 Recipes

With Ingredients Detail

- Lipstick
- Mascara
- Face Mist
- Blush
- Eyeliner
- Eyeshadow
- Nail Polish
- Body Glitter
- Foundation
- Primer
- Highlighter
- Face Powder

Shahaan Merchant

Start Your Own Homemade Organic Cosmetics Brand 110 Recipes

. . . .

By

Shahaan Merchant

Copyright

Disclaimer

The information provided in this book is for educational and informational purposes only. The recipes, instructions, and formulations shared are based on research and experience but are not guaranteed to be error-free, accurate, or suitable for all individuals or circumstances.While every effort has been made to ensure accuracy, the authors and publishers cannot be held responsible for any adverse reactions, accidents, or damages that may arise from the use, misuse, or application of the information contained herein.

Readers understand and acknowledge that the creation, application, or use of homemade products described in this book carries inherent risks. The authors, publishers, and affiliated parties do not assume any responsibility or liability for the accuracy, completeness, suitability, or outcomes resulting from the utilization of the information presented herein.

Furthermore, the authors and publishers disclaim any responsibility for:

Allergic reactions, skin irritations, or adverse health effects resulting from the use of homemade products, as individual sensitivities vary.

Accidents, damages, or injuries incurred during the production, application, or storage of homemade products.

Any inaccuracies, omissions, or errors in the recipes, formulations, or instructions provided.

Readers are strongly advised to:

Conduct patch tests and seek professional advice before using any homemade products, especially if they have known allergies, sensitivities, or health conditions.

Perform thorough research, including cross-referencing multiple sources, to ensure the safety, suitability, and legality of ingredients and methods used.

Adhere to safety guidelines, including proper storage, handling of ingredients, and compliance with local regulations and laws concerning product manufacturing and distribution.

By using the information in this book, readers agree to hold harmless the authors, publishers, and affiliates from any liability, claims, damages, or expenses that may arise directly or indirectly from the use or misuse of the provided information.

Table of Contents

Nail Polish

Nail Polish Remover

Primer

Foundation

Concealer

Blush

Eyeliner & Highlighter

Bronzer

Setting Spray

Face Powder

Eyeshadow

Face Mist

DIY ORGANIC ROSEWATER Face Mist: Refreshing Floral Elixir for Your Skin

DIY Organic Green Tea Face Mist: Revitalize Your Skin with Nature's Goodness

DIY Organic Lavender Face Mist: Nourish Your Skin with Nature's Serenity

It was January 19th, 1992, and I found myself in my favorite cosmetic shop, surrounded by vibrant colors and promises of glamour. There it was, a beautiful makeup kit that seemed straight out of a dream. I could picture the smoothness of the eyeshadows and the radiance of the blush. But as my eyes glanced at the price tag, my heart sank. It was beyond what my pocket money could stretch to.

I thought about asking Dad for extra money, but then I remembered the growing pile of bills that he had to deal with. I couldn't add to his worries. So, reluctantly, I put the makeup kit back on the shelf. Even a simple lipstick felt like a luxury I couldn't afford. Disappointed, I left the shop empty-handed.

On my way home, feeling dejected, I bought a fashion magazine that featured stunning models adorned in glamorous makeup. Maybe it was a way to capture a bit of that magic within its glossy pages.

Back home, Mom had prepared a delicious dinner, and as we sat together, laughter filled the air. But my mind kept wandering back to the unreachable makeup kit. Later, when I finally went to bed, the magazine in my hands caught my attention.

As I flipped through the pages, I found myself in awe of the flawless models and their perfect makeup. Then, almost hidden within these glamorous images, I stumbled upon a section about homemade cosmetics. Recipes to create makeup from everyday ingredients! Could it be real?

I was drawn to a simple recipe for homemade lip balm. The ingredients were kitchen staples - coconut oil, beeswax, and a touch of essential oil for fragrance. Hope flickered within me. Could this be my solution?

As I lay in bed that night, I couldn't sleep. Excitement bubbled within me, and I kept glancing at the clock, waiting for the morning to arrive. I was on a mission - a mission to create my very own homemade cosmetics. The recipes I had stumbled upon in that magazine felt like a treasure map leading to a world of possibilities.

Morning finally broke, and I practically leaped out of bed, eager to start my quest. I hurried through my morning routine, barely able to contain my excitement. Grabbing my jacket and some cash, I practically skipped out the door, heading straight to the local store.

Entering the shop, I was like a kid in a candy store, but instead of sweets, I was surrounded by rows of ingredients waiting to be transformed into beauty treasures. I grabbed coconut oil, beeswax, and a small bottle of lavender essential oil, feeling a rush of exhilaration as I placed them in my basket.

Back home, I cleared a spot in the kitchen, laying out my newly acquired ingredients. I carefully read and reread the recipe for homemade lip balm, making sure I understood each step. With a mix of excitement and nerves, I began melting the beeswax on the stove.

The kitchen soon filled with the sweet aroma of beeswax, and as I added the coconut oil, a sense of anticipation filled the air. But as I poured the mixture into the containers, it was a bit of a mess. Wax dripped, oil splattered, and I ended up with more on the counter than in the containers.

Disappointment tried to creep in, but I reminded myself that every mistake is a lesson. I cleaned up the kitchen, determined not to give up. I readjusted my approach, measured the ingredients with even more care, and gave it another shot.

This time, as the beeswax and coconut oil blended together, I could feel something different in the air. It was like the ingredients were harmonizing perfectly. Adding a few drops of the lavender essential oil, the kitchen filled with a delicate, soothing scent.

With a steady hand, I poured the mixture into the containers, and this time, it went smoothly. The lip balm looked perfect, glistening in its little pots. I couldn't contain my joy—I had done it! I had made my very own homemade lip balm.

I celebrated by dancing around the kitchen, laughing out loud in pure happiness. I held the little pots of lip balm like precious gems, feeling an immense sense of accomplishment. Applying the lip balm to my lips, I felt a rush of pride. It wasn't just a lip balm; it was a symbol of my determination and the beginning of my homemade cosmetics journey.

That day, I shared my success with my family, and their smiles mirrored my own happiness. It wasn't just about the lip balm; it was about the journey of discovery, the joy of creation, and the realization that sometimes, the most beautiful things are made right in our own kitchens.

I was super excited about it, you know? But boy, did things turn out different from what I expected!

After I made that lip balm, I felt like I'd found a treasure. I showed it to my friends, all giddy and proud. But instead of cheering me on, they made fun of me! Can you believe it? They laughed at my homemade lip balm and didn't take it seriously at all. One friend even called it "pathetic."

Man, did that hurt. I put my heart into making that lip balm, and they just brushed it off like it was nothing. It was a bit discouraging, to be honest. I thought, maybe I was just fooling myself, thinking I could create something worthwhile.

But you know, life has a funny way of surprising you. Even though my friends weren't interested, my aunt, bless her heart, was always up for trying new things. So, one day, she saw that lip balm sitting on my dresser and asked if she could give it a try.

I was hesitant at first, thinking she might dislike it too, or worse, make fun of me like my friends did. But she insisted, saying she trusted my creativity. So, I handed it over, feeling a bit nervous.

Days passed, and I kinda forgot about that whole lip balm thing amidst the teasing from my friends. Then one day, my aunt called me over, looking excited. She told me she had been using my homemade lip balm and, guess what? She loved it! She said it was amazing, and it made her lips feel soft and hydrated.

I was surprised, to say the least. I mean, I made it just for fun, not expecting anyone to actually like it! But my aunt's praise gave me a bit of hope, you know? It was like a little spark in my heart, reminding me that maybe there was something special about that lip balm after all.

It didn't stop there, though. My aunt started telling her friends about it. And before I knew it, they all wanted to try it too! They loved it just as much as she did. Suddenly, that lip balm that my friends called "pathetic" was getting some serious attention.

Word spread, and people from the neighborhood wanted to get their hands on it. I started making more batches, experimenting with different scents and textures. It was wild! My homemade lip balm was becoming a hit!

Funny how things turned out, right? From being laughed at by my friends to having my homemade creation praised by my aunt and loved by so many others. It taught me something valuable: sometimes, the people who believe in you might not be the ones you expect. And sometimes, the things you create for fun can turn into something truly amazing.

I wanted to try different things, experiment with makeup, and make my own skincare products. So, I turned to magazines hoping to find some cool recipes. But you know what the problem was? Those magazines only had like two or three recipes per month, and that just wasn't enough for my curious mind.

Then, it hit me. My dad's friend actually worked in a cosmetics factory! I thought he might have some insider knowledge, you know, some secret formulas or something. So, I mustered up the courage and asked Dad if he could introduce me to his friend.

But Dad wasn't too keen on the idea. He said his friend might make fun of me or something. I felt disappointed; I really wanted to explore this world of cosmetics. So, I didn't give up. I bugged Dad, convinced him that I just wanted to learn and try new things. After a lot of pestering, he finally agreed to introduce me to his friend.

When I met Dad's friend from the cosmetics factory, I was a bit nervous. I thought he might laugh at my curiosity or say that making cosmetics was too complicated for a girl like me. But you know what? He was actually pretty cool about it. He listened to my questions, and instead of giving me complex chemical formulas, he shared some basic principles of making skincare products. He even gave me a few simple recipes to start with.

Now, here's the twist. Instead of using all those chemicals that I couldn't even pronounce, I decided to take a different route. I wanted to keep it natural, you know? So, I used ingredients from my kitchen—coconut oil, honey, oats, and other stuff that I knew were good for the skin.

At first, it was a bit of trial and error. Some of my creations were total disasters. I remember this one face mask I made that turned into a gooey mess and made my face look like I'd dipped it in mud! But hey, I didn't let that discourage me.

I kept experimenting, tweaking the recipes, adjusting the quantities, and slowly, things started to work. I made my own face scrubs, masks, and even a simple moisturizer that smelled like heaven.

When I finally nailed a recipe, I was over the moon! I celebrated by treating myself to a little spa day at home using my homemade products. It was like magic—my skin felt amazing, and I felt like I'd cracked the code to my own little beauty secrets.

It taught me something important, you know? Sometimes, you don't need fancy or expensive things to make something special. Natural ingredients and a dash of curiosity can create wonders.

Fast forward 25 years, and something amazing happened.

One day, my son, a little rascal, comes up to me holding this dusty, messy book. It was almost falling apart! As I looked closer, I realized it was my makeup recipes book from all those years ago. I was speechless; my heart skipped a beat. Tears welled up in my eyes as I leafed through those worn-out pages. Those were the very recipes that kickstarted everything for me.

I held that book close to my heart and thought about where life had taken me. From that girl who couldn't afford fancy cosmetics to building a successful brand.

It was a story that began with a girl who couldn't afford expensive cosmetics and turned into something beyond her wildest dreams—a story that I now had the chance to share with the world.

Hi, I'm Shahaan, author of this book. As I sit here, penning down these thoughts, I can't help but reflect on the power of stories. Have you ever been inspired by a tale of courage, of someone taking a leap of faith and creating something extraordinary out of sheer passion? That's the kind of story that fuels my belief in the potential of every individual, especially the incredible women out there.

The story you just read about the girl passionate about cosmetics, facing limitations but finding a way to create her own path—well, that's just one among countless tales scattered across the globe. There are stories hidden behind some of the top brands we admire today, stories of people who were perhaps average or even below average in the eyes of the world. But they dared to take a courageous step, they started something small, and now, their brands stand as status symbols.

I truly believe in the power of womanhood, in the strength, resilience, and limitless potential that each of you possesses. It takes just one product, one idea, to spark the journey of a successful business and brand. And you know what the secret ingredient is? Action.

I'm a true believer in woman empowerment. I believe that behind every successful woman is a story of determination, of overcoming obstacles, and of rising against the odds. I'm here to tell you that you, yes, you reading this, have that same potential within you.

You might think, "But what can I do? I'm just an ordinary person." But let me tell you, every big success starts with a small step, a courageous decision to try. It's about believing in yourself, your abilities, and your dreams. You have a treasure trove of creativity within you, waiting to be unleashed.

So, my dear ladies, it's time to awaken that courage within. Take that step. Start your own brand, your own journey. Let your passion be your guide. Don't let limitations or doubts hold you back. Embrace the power of your dreams, and remember, you have the ability to turn those dreams into reality.

Believe in yourself, take that leap, and watch as your story unfolds, inspiring others along the way. Because when a woman believes in herself, she can move mountains. You have the potential to create, to inspire, and to leave a mark on the world. And I'll be here, cheering you on every step of the way.

Here's to you, to your courage, and to the incredible journey of creating something beautiful out of your passion. Go on, wonder ladies, let your brilliance shine!

I wanted to have a heart-to-heart with you, just like friends chatting over a cup of coffee. You see, this book, well, it's more than just a bunch of instructions on paper. It's a treasure trove, a guide to a world where courage meets creativity.

This book is a call to all the Wonder Women out there, to all the housewives who might think they don't have the courage to dream big. I'm here to tell you that you do! It's about starting small but thinking big. It's about taking these recipes, these little nuggets of gold, and turning them into something magical.

It was about belief, about having the courage to take that first step. I wanted to inspire others, especially all the incredible women out there, to take that leap of faith. You don't need a big investment or a fancy setup to start something amazing. All you need is a bit of courage and a whole lot of determination.

So, to all of you who will read this book and embark on your own journey of homemade cosmetics, remember this: You are capable of incredible things. Dream big, start small, and don't be afraid to take that leap. You have the power within you to turn these recipes into something truly special.

I'm willing to create a series of recipes in different products, just to make sure you have all the tools for success. I know how it feels to crave that guidance, that little push in the right direction. Let's make this book not just a sale but a sensation! Let's spread the joy of homemade cosmetics far and wide. Because in the end, it's not just about the products; it's about the community, the support, and the shared passion for beauty that brings us all together.

So, to all of you holding this book, remember, you're not alone on this journey. Reach out, let's connect, and let's create something amazing together. Here's to dreams, to courage, and to the power of homemade organic beauty!

With Lots of Love & Warm Regards,

Shahaan Merchant

Ingredients

Understanding the Basics

Each ingredient in your recipes serves a specific purpose. They are carefully selected for their natural benefits. For instance:

- Coconut Oil: Provides hydration and acts as a base for many recipes.
- Shea Butter: Rich in vitamins, it moisturizes and soothes the skin.
- Essential Oils: Offer various aromas and possess unique properties like calming or rejuvenating effects.
- Clay Powders: Known for cleansing and detoxifying the skin.

Why These Ingredients?

THESE INGREDIENTS ARE chosen for their gentle yet effective nature. Coconut oil and shea butter work as excellent bases due to their moisturizing properties. Essential oils offer fragrance while also delivering specific benefits for the skin or hair. Clay powders are used for cleansing and purifying.

Tools You'll Need

TO BEGIN YOUR COSMETIC journey, gather these basic tools:

- Mixing Bowls: For blending ingredients.
- Spatulas: To mix and apply the products.
- Glass Jars/Containers: For storing the final products.
- Measuring Spoons/Cups: For accurate measurements.

Methods

Home Version

GATHER INGREDIENTS: Measure out the required quantities.
Mixing: Combine the ingredients as per the recipe instructions.
Storage: Pour the mixture into suitable containers.

Usage: Apply or use the product as directed.

Commercial Version

SCALING UP: INCREASE the ingredient quantities proportionally.
Quality Control: Ensure consistency and quality across batches.
Packaging: Invest in professional-looking packaging for retail.

Additional Tips

- EXPERIMENTATION: Don't be afraid to try new ingredient combinations.
  - Labeling: Always label your creations with ingredients and dates.
  - Research: Keep exploring new ingredients and their benefits.

Caution

- ALLERGIES: BE CAUTIOUS of known allergies to certain ingredients.
  - Patch Test: Before full application, test on a small skin area.

Shelf Life

THE SHELF LIFE VARIES based on ingredients used. Typically, products can last from a few weeks to several months. Always note the expiration dates and store them properly.

Packaging Tips

- AIRTIGHT CONTAINERS: Prevents contamination and extends shelf life.
  - Attractive Labeling: Clear and appealing labels attract customers.
  - Eco-Friendly: Consider sustainable packaging options.

Unique Selling Proposition (USP)

THE BEAUTY OF YOUR homemade organic cosmetics lies in their natural ingredients. Highlight the purity, eco-friendliness, and unique blends that commercial products often lack. Emphasize the handmade, personal touch that customers love.

This book is your gateway to creating natural, organic cosmetics. Experiment, explore, and most importantly, have fun crafting your brand!

Ingredients

1. Beeswax (1/2 teaspoon)

Beeswax helps the mascara maintain its shape and texture while being gentle on the skin. It also aids in creating a smooth application.

2. Coconut Oil (1 teaspoon)

COCONUT OIL MOISTURIZES the lashes, preventing them from becoming brittle. It also helps in giving the mascara a smooth consistency.

3. Charcoal Powder (1/4 teaspoon)

CHARCOAL POWDER PROVIDES the intense black color naturally without any harmful additives. It's gentle and safe for use around the eyes.

4. Aloe Vera Gel (1/2 teaspoon)

ALOE VERA GEL NOURISHES the lashes and soothes the delicate skin around the eyes. It also contributes to the mascara's smooth application.

5. Vitamin E Oil (2-3 drops)

VITAMIN E OIL ACTS as a natural preservative, extending the shelf life of the mascara while also nourishing the lashes.

Tools Required

- SMALL SAUCEPAN
  - Glass or stainless steel bowl
  - Spoon for mixing
  - Empty mascara tube or container
  - Small funnel (optional)

Method

Homemade Version

- PREPARE INGREDIENTS: Gather all the ingredients in their measured quantities.
  - Double Boiling: Fill the small saucepan with water and place it on low heat. Put the glass or stainless steel bowl in the saucepan, making sure it doesn't touch the water.
  - Mix Ingredients: Add beeswax and coconut oil to the bowl. Stir gently until they melt together.
  - Add Charcoal and Aloe Vera: Once melted, remove the bowl from heat and add charcoal powder, aloe vera gel, and vitamin E oil. Mix well until you achieve a smooth, consistent mixture.
  - Transfer to Container: Carefully pour the mixture into the mascara tube or container using a small funnel or by pouring directly if the opening is wide enough. Allow it to cool and solidify before use.

Additional Tips

- *Texture Adjustments:* If the mascara seems too thick, add a tiny amount of coconut oil. For a thinner consistency, add more aloe vera gel.
  - *Application:* Use a clean mascara wand for application. Wipe off excess product to avoid clumps.
  - *Storage:* Keep the mascara in a cool, dry place away from direct sunlight.

Caution

- ALWAYS PERFORM A patch test before applying any homemade cosmetics, especially around the eyes, to ensure you don't have any allergic reactions.

Commercial Version

TO PRODUCE THIS MASCARA on a larger scale for commercial purposes, you may need to alter the recipe slightly and consider adding natural preservatives to extend shelf life. You can also enhance the formula by incorporating ingredients like castor oil for lash nourishment and beeswax for a smoother application.

Ingredients for Commercial Version

- CASTOR OIL (1/2 teaspoon)
  - Natural Preservative (As per manufacturer's guidelines)

Shelf Life & Packaging Tips

THE HOMEMADE MASCARA can last for about 3-6 months if stored properly. For commercial use, with added preservatives, it can have a longer shelf life—around 6-12 months. Consider using air-tight, dark-colored containers to preserve the mascara and protect it from light exposure.

Unique Selling Proposition (USP)

HIGHLIGHT THE MASCARA'S natural ingredients, its nourishing properties for lashes, and its gentle formula suitable for sensitive eyes.

This homemade organic black mascara is a gentle, nourishing option for those looking to embrace natural cosmetics. Whether for personal use or commercial production, it provides a safe and effective alternative to conventional mascaras.

Organic Brown Mascara with Cocoa Powder

Ingredients

1. Beeswax (1/2 teaspoon)

Beeswax helps maintain the mascara's consistency and structure while being gentle on the skin. It aids in achieving a smooth application.

2. Coconut Oil (1 teaspoon)

COCONUT OIL PROVIDES moisture to the lashes, preventing them from becoming brittle. It contributes to the mascara's smooth texture.

3. Cocoa Powder (1/4 teaspoon)

COCOA POWDER ADDS A natural brown color without any harmful additives. It's safe for use around the eyes and provides a beautiful, subtle brown hue.

4. Aloe Vera Gel (1/2 teaspoon)

ALOE VERA GEL NOURISHES and soothes the lashes and delicate skin around the eyes. It helps in the smooth application of the mascara.

5. Vitamin E Oil (2-3 drops)

VITAMIN E OIL ACTS as a natural preservative, extending the mascara's shelf life while also nourishing the lashes.

Tools Required

- SMALL SAUCEPAN
  - Glass or stainless steel bowl
  - Spoon for mixing
  - Empty mascara tube or container
  - Small funnel (optional)

Method

Homemade Version

- PREPARE INGREDIENTS: Measure out all the ingredients accurately.
- Double Boiling: Fill the small saucepan with water and put it on low heat. Place the glass or stainless steel bowl in the saucepan, ensuring it doesn't touch the water.
- Mix Ingredients: Add beeswax and coconut oil to the bowl. Stir gently until they melt together.
- Incorporate Cocoa and Aloe Vera: Remove the bowl from heat once melted. Add cocoa powder, aloe vera gel, and vitamin E oil. Mix thoroughly until a smooth, consistent mixture forms.
- Transfer to Container: Carefully pour the mixture into the mascara tube or container. Allow it to cool and solidify before use.

Additional Tips

- *Texture Adjustments:* Add a small amount of coconut oil if the mascara appears too thick. For a thinner consistency, increase the amount of aloe vera gel.
- *Application:* Use a clean mascara wand for application. Wipe off excess product to prevent clumping.
- *Storage:* Store the mascara in a cool, dry place away from direct sunlight.

Caution

- ALWAYS CONDUCT A patch test before applying any homemade cosmetics around the eyes to check for allergic reactions.

Commercial Version

FOR COMMERCIAL PRODUCTION, slight adjustments may be necessary. Consider adding natural preservatives to prolong shelf life. Additionally, enhancing the formula with ingredients like castor oil for lash nourishment could be beneficial.

Ingredients for Commercial Version

- CASTOR OIL (1/2 teaspoon)
  - Natural Preservative (As per manufacturer's guidelines)

Shelf Life & Packaging Tips

THE HOMEMADE BROWN mascara, if stored properly, can last for approximately 3-6 months. With added natural preservatives for commercial use, it may have a longer shelf life of around 6-12 months. Using airtight, dark-colored containers helps preserve the mascara and protect it from light exposure.

Unique Selling Proposition (USP)

HIGHLIGHT THE MASCARA'S natural ingredients, its ability to nourish lashes, and its gentle, organic formula ideal for sensitive eyes.

This homemade organic brown mascara enriched with cocoa powder offers a subtle, natural-looking brown tint. Whether for personal use or potential commercial production, it provides a safe and effective alternative to conventional mascaras.

Organic Almond Oil Mascara

Ingredients

1. Beeswax (1/2 teaspoon)

Beeswax helps maintain the mascara's consistency and structure while being gentle on the skin. It aids in achieving a smooth application.

2. Almond Oil (1 teaspoon)

ALMOND OIL NOURISHES and strengthens lashes, promoting their growth. It also provides a glossy finish and helps condition the delicate skin around the eyes.

3. Activated Charcoal Powder (1/4 teaspoon)

ACTIVATED CHARCOAL powder gives a deep black color naturally without any harmful additives. It's safe for use around the eyes and provides an intense hue.

4. Aloe Vera Gel (1/2 teaspoon)

ALOE VERA GEL SOOTHES the lashes and the sensitive skin around the eyes. It contributes to the mascara's smooth application and adds moisture.

5. Vitamin E Oil (2-3 drops)

VITAMIN E OIL ACTS as a natural preservative, extending the mascara's shelf life while nourishing the lashes.

Tools Required

- SMALL SAUCEPAN
  - Glass or stainless steel bowl
  - Spoon for mixing
  - Empty mascara tube or container

- Small funnel (optional)

Method

Homemade Version

- PREPARE INGREDIENTS: Measure out all the ingredients accurately.
- Double Boiling: Fill the small saucepan with water and place it on low heat. Put the glass or stainless steel bowl in the saucepan, ensuring it doesn't touch the water.
- Mix Ingredients: Add beeswax and almond oil to the bowl. Stir gently until they melt together.
- Incorporate Charcoal and Aloe Vera: Once melted, remove the bowl from heat. Add activated charcoal powder, aloe vera gel, and vitamin E oil. Mix thoroughly until a smooth, consistent mixture forms.
- Transfer to Container: Carefully pour the mixture into the mascara tube or container. Allow it to cool and solidify before use.

Additional Tips

- *Texture Adjustments:* If the mascara appears too thick, add a small amount of almond oil. For a thinner consistency, increase the amount of aloe vera gel.
- *Application:* Use a clean mascara wand for application. Wipe off excess product to prevent clumping.
- *Storage:* Store the mascara in a cool, dry place away from direct sunlight.

Caution

- ALWAYS PERFORM A patch test before applying any homemade cosmetics around the eyes to check for allergic reactions.

Commercial Version

FOR COMMERCIAL PRODUCTION, consider incorporating natural preservatives to prolong shelf life and enhancing the formula with additional lash-nourishing ingredients like castor oil or jojoba oil.

Ingredients for Commercial Version

- CASTOR OIL OR JOJOBA Oil (1/2 teaspoon)
  - Natural Preservative (As per manufacturer's guidelines)

Shelf Life & Packaging Tips

THE HOMEMADE ALMOND oil mascara, if stored properly, can last for approximately 3-6 months. With added natural preservatives for commercial use, it may have a shelf life of around 6-12 months. Use airtight, dark-colored containers to preserve the mascara and shield it from light exposure.

Unique Selling Proposition (USP)

HIGHLIGHT THE MASCARA'S natural ingredients, emphasizing its lash-nourishing properties and its gentle, organic formula suitable for sensitive eyes.

This homemade organic almond oil mascara provides nourishment and intense color, promoting healthy lashes. Whether for personal use or potential commercial production, it offers a safe and effective alternative to conventional mascaras.

Ingredients

1. Beeswax (1/2 teaspoon)

Beeswax helps the mascara hold its shape and texture, contributing to voluminous lashes. It ensures a smooth application without clumping.

2. Coconut Oil (1 teaspoon)

COCONUT OIL MOISTURIZES and nourishes the lashes, preventing breakage and promoting volume. It also aids in achieving a creamy consistency for the mascara.

3. Activated Charcoal Powder (1/4 teaspoon)

ACTIVATED CHARCOAL provides a deep black color naturally, enhancing the mascara's intensity without any harmful additives.

4. Aloe Vera Gel (1/2 teaspoon)

ALOE VERA GEL NOURISHES and strengthens lashes, promoting their growth and adding volume. It also helps in the smooth application of the mascara.

5. Castor Oil (2-3 drops)

CASTOR OIL SUPPORTS lash growth and thickness, contributing to voluminous lashes.

Tools Required

- SMALL SAUCEPAN
  - Glass or stainless steel bowl
  - Spoon for mixing
  - Empty mascara tube or container

- Small funnel (optional)

Method

Homemade Version

- PREPARE INGREDIENTS: Measure all the ingredients accurately.
- Double Boiling: Fill the small saucepan with water and heat it on low. Place the glass or stainless steel bowl in the saucepan, ensuring it doesn't touch the water.
- Mix Ingredients: Add beeswax and coconut oil to the bowl. Stir gently until they melt together.
- Add Charcoal, Aloe Vera, and Castor Oil: Remove the bowl from heat once melted. Add activated charcoal powder, aloe vera gel, and castor oil. Mix thoroughly until achieving a smooth, consistent mixture.
- Transfer to Container: Carefully pour the mixture into the mascara tube or container. Let it cool and solidify before use.

Additional Tips

- *Texture Adjustments:* Increase coconut oil for a smoother texture or add a touch more charcoal for a darker hue.
- *Application:* Use a clean mascara wand. Wipe excess product to avoid clumps.
- *Storage:* Keep the mascara in a cool, dry place away from direct sunlight.

Caution

- ALWAYS PERFORM A patch test before applying any homemade cosmetics around the eyes to check for allergic reactions.

Commercial Version

FOR COMMERCIAL PRODUCTION, incorporating natural preservatives may be necessary to extend shelf life. Consider enhancing the formula with ingredients like vitamin E oil for additional nourishment.

Ingredients for Commercial Version

- VITAMIN E OIL (2-3 drops)
  - Natural Preservative (As per manufacturer's guidelines)

Shelf Life & Packaging Tips

THE HOMEMADE VOLUMIZING mascara, if stored properly, can last for around 3-6 months. With added natural preservatives for commercial use, it might have a shelf life of approximately 6-12 months. Dark-colored, airtight containers are ideal for preserving the mascara and protecting it from light exposure.

Unique Selling Proposition (USP)

HIGHLIGHT THE MASCARA'S volumizing properties, emphasizing its natural, organic ingredients promoting lash growth and thickness. The mascara provides a safe and effective alternative to conventional volumizing mascaras.

Ingredients

1. Beeswax (1/2 teaspoon)

Beeswax helps the mascara maintain its shape and texture, preventing clumping and aiding in a smooth application. It contributes to elongating the lashes.

2. Coconut Oil (1 teaspoon)

COCONUT OIL MOISTURIZES and nourishes lashes, preventing breakage and promoting their length. It also helps in achieving a creamy texture for the mascara.

3. Castor Oil (1/2 teaspoon)

CASTOR OIL SUPPORTS lash growth, making them thicker and longer over time. It contributes to the lengthening effect of the mascara.

4. Activated Charcoal Powder (1/4 teaspoon)

ACTIVATED CHARCOAL provides a deep black color naturally without any harmful additives. It intensifies the mascara's hue while being safe for use around the eyes.

5. Aloe Vera Gel (1/2 teaspoon)

ALOE VERA GEL NOURISHES lashes and soothes the delicate skin around the eyes. It helps in achieving a smooth application and contributes to the mascara's lengthening effect.

6. Vitamin E Oil (2-3 drops)

VITAMIN E OIL ACTS as a natural preservative, extending the mascara's shelf life while nourishing and strengthening lashes.

Tools Required

- SMALL SAUCEPAN
  - Glass or stainless steel bowl
  - Spoon for mixing
  - Empty mascara tube or container
  - Small funnel (optional)

Method

Homemade Version

- PREPARE INGREDIENTS: Measure all the ingredients accurately.
  - Double Boiling: Fill the small saucepan with water and heat it on low. Place the glass or stainless steel bowl in the saucepan, ensuring it doesn't touch the water.
  - Mix Ingredients: Add beeswax and coconut oil to the bowl. Stir gently until they melt together.
  - Incorporate Charcoal, Aloe Vera, Castor Oil, and Vitamin E: Remove the bowl from heat once melted. Add activated charcoal powder, aloe vera gel, castor oil, and vitamin E oil. Mix thoroughly until a smooth, consistent mixture forms.
  - Transfer to Container: Carefully pour the mixture into the mascara tube or container. Allow it to cool and solidify before use.

Additional Tips

- *Texture Adjustments:* Add a bit more coconut oil for a smoother texture. Increase charcoal powder for a darker hue.
  - *Application:* Use a clean mascara wand. Wipe off excess product to prevent clumps.
  - *Storage:* Keep the mascara in a cool, dry place away from direct sunlight.

Caution

- ALWAYS CONDUCT A patch test before applying any homemade cosmetics around the eyes to check for allergic reactions.

Commercial Version

FOR COMMERCIAL PRODUCTION, consider adding natural preservatives to extend shelf life. Enhance the formula with additional ingredients like argan oil for added nourishment and lengthening properties.

Ingredients for Commercial Version

- ARGAN OIL (1/2 TEASPOON)
  - Natural Preservative (As per manufacturer's guidelines)

Shelf Life & Packaging Tips

THE HOMEMADE LENGTHENING mascara, if stored properly, can last for around 3-6 months. With added natural preservatives for commercial use, it might have a shelf life of approximately 6-12 months. Opt for airtight, dark-colored containers to preserve the mascara and shield it from light exposure.

Unique Selling Proposition (USP)

HIGHLIGHT THE MASCARA'S lengthening properties, emphasizing its natural, organic ingredients that promote lash growth and length. This mascara provides a safe and effective alternative to conventional lengthening mascaras.

Ingredients

1. Beeswax (1/2 teaspoon)

Beeswax helps the mascara maintain its structure and texture, ensuring smooth application and color retention. It's crucial for holding the colorful pigments together.

2. Coconut Oil (1 teaspoon)

COCONUT OIL MOISTURIZES lashes, preventing them from drying out and breaking. It also contributes to the mascara's creamy texture and helps spread the pigments evenly.

3. Colored Natural Pigments (1/4 teaspoon each)

CHOOSE ORGANIC, NATURAL pigments according to the desired color—spirulina powder for green, beetroot powder for red, turmeric for yellow, or cocoa powder for brown.

4. Aloe Vera Gel (1/2 teaspoon)

ALOE VERA GEL SOOTHES the lashes and the sensitive skin around the eyes. It helps in achieving a smooth application and contributes to the mascara's overall texture.

5. Vitamin E Oil (2-3 drops)

VITAMIN E OIL ACTS as a natural preservative, extending the mascara's shelf life while nourishing the lashes.

Tools Required

- SMALL SAUCEPAN
  - Glass or stainless steel bowl

- Spoon for mixing
- Empty mascara tube or container
- Small funnel (optional)

Method

Homemade Version

- PREPARE INGREDIENTS: Measure all the ingredients accurately.
- Double Boiling: Fill the small saucepan with water and heat it on low. Place the glass or stainless steel bowl in the saucepan, ensuring it doesn't touch the water.
- Mix Ingredients: Add beeswax and coconut oil to the bowl. Stir gently until they melt together.
- Incorporate Natural Pigments, Aloe Vera, and Vitamin E: Remove the bowl from heat once melted. Add the chosen natural pigments, aloe vera gel, and vitamin E oil. Mix thoroughly until a smooth, consistent mixture forms.
- Transfer to Container: Carefully pour the colored mixture into the mascara tube or container. Allow it to cool and solidify before use.

Additional Tips

- *Pigment Intensity:* Adjust the amount of natural pigments to achieve the desired color intensity.
- *Texture Adjustments:* Add more coconut oil for a smoother texture or adjust beeswax for a firmer consistency.
- *Application:* Use a clean mascara wand for application. Wipe off excess product to avoid clumping.
- *Storage:* Keep the mascara in a cool, dry place away from direct sunlight.

Caution

- ALWAYS PERFORM A patch test before applying any homemade cosmetics around the eyes to check for allergic reactions.

Commercial Version

FOR COMMERCIAL PRODUCTION, incorporating natural preservatives may be necessary to extend shelf life. Additionally, consider enhancing the formula with ingredients like mica powder for shimmer or additional natural pigments for a broader color range.

Ingredients for Commercial Version

- MICA POWDER (FOR shimmer)
  - Natural Preservative (As per manufacturer's guidelines)

Shelf Life & Packaging Tips

THE HOMEMADE COLORFUL mascara, if stored properly, can last for around 3-6 months. With added natural preservatives for commercial use, it might have a shelf life of approximately 6-12 months. Opt for airtight, dark-colored containers to preserve the mascara and shield it from light exposure.

Unique Selling Proposition (USP)

HIGHLIGHT THE MASCARA'S vibrant, organic colors, emphasizing its natural, safe ingredients that offer a playful and unique way to enhance lashes. This mascara provides a safe and creative alternative to conventional makeup choices.

Ingredients

1. Beeswax (1/2 teaspoon)

Beeswax provides structure and texture to the mascara, preventing clumping and aiding in a smooth application. It helps the fibers adhere to lashes.

2. Coconut Oil (1 teaspoon)

COCONUT OIL MOISTURIZES and conditions lashes, preventing breakage. It also helps in achieving a creamy texture for the mascara.

3. Plant-Based Fibers (1/4 teaspoon)

CHOOSE ORGANIC, PLANT-based fibers like cotton or silk. These fibers help add length and volume to lashes, creating a fuller appearance.

4. Aloe Vera Gel (1/2 teaspoon)

ALOE VERA GEL SOOTHES the lashes and delicate eye skin. It contributes to the mascara's smooth application and overall texture.

5. Vitamin E Oil (2-3 drops)

VITAMIN E OIL ACTS as a natural preservative, extending the mascara's shelf life while nourishing and strengthening lashes.

Tools Required

- SMALL SAUCEPAN
  - Glass or stainless steel bowl
  - Spoon for mixing
  - Empty mascara tube or container
  - Small funnel (optional)

Method

Homemade Version

- PREPARE INGREDIENTS: Measure out all the ingredients accurately.
- Double Boiling: Fill the small saucepan with water and heat it on low. Place the glass or stainless steel bowl in the saucepan, ensuring it doesn't touch the water.
- Mix Ingredients: Add beeswax and coconut oil to the bowl. Stir gently until they melt together.
- Incorporate Plant-Based Fibers, Aloe Vera, and Vitamin E: Remove the bowl from heat once melted. Add plant-based fibers, aloe vera gel, and vitamin E oil. Mix thoroughly until a smooth, consistent mixture forms.
- Transfer to Container: Carefully pour the fiber-infused mixture into the mascara tube or container. Allow it to cool and solidify before use.

Additional Tips

- *Fiber Intensity:* Adjust the amount of plant-based fibers for desired lash length and volume.
- *Texture Adjustments:* Add more coconut oil for a smoother texture or adjust beeswax for a firmer consistency.
- *Application:* Use a clean mascara wand for application. Wipe off excess product to avoid clumps.
- *Storage:* Keep the mascara in a cool, dry place away from direct sunlight.

Caution

- ALWAYS PERFORM A patch test before applying any homemade cosmetics around the eyes to check for allergic reactions.

Commercial Version

FOR COMMERCIAL PRODUCTION, consider adding natural preservatives to extend shelf life. Enhance the formula with additional lash-nourishing ingredients like castor oil or argan oil for added benefits.

Ingredients for Commercial Version

- CASTOR OIL OR ARGAN Oil (1/2 teaspoon)
  - Natural Preservative (As per manufacturer's guidelines)

Shelf Life & Packaging Tips

THE HOMEMADE FIBER mascara, if stored properly, can last for around 3-6 months. With added natural preservatives for commercial use, it might have a shelf life of approximately 6-12 months. Use airtight, dark-colored containers for preservation and to protect the mascara from light exposure.

Unique Selling Proposition (USP)

HIGHLIGHT THE MASCARA'S ability to add length and volume using organic, plant-based fibers. Emphasize its natural, gentle formula that promotes fuller-looking lashes without synthetic additives. This mascara provides a safe and effective alternative to conventional fiber mascaras.

Ingredients

1. Beeswax (1/2 teaspoon)

Beeswax helps maintain the mascara's consistency and prevents clumping by providing structure. It ensures a smooth application.

2. Coconut Oil (1 teaspoon)

COCONUT OIL MOISTURIZES lashes, preventing them from sticking together and causing clumps. It also contributes to the mascara's smooth texture.

3. Arrowroot Powder (1/4 teaspoon)

ARROWROOT POWDER ACTS as a natural thickening agent, preventing clumping and giving the mascara a smooth, clump-free consistency.

4. Aloe Vera Gel (1/2 teaspoon)

ALOE VERA GEL SOOTHES the lashes and the delicate skin around the eyes, contributing to a smooth application and preventing clumping.

5. Vitamin E Oil (2-3 drops)

VITAMIN E OIL ACTS as a natural preservative, extending the mascara's shelf life while nourishing the lashes.

Tools Required

- SMALL SAUCEPAN
  - Glass or stainless steel bowl
  - Spoon for mixing
  - Empty mascara tube or container

- Small funnel (optional)

Method

Homemade Version

- PREPARE INGREDIENTS: Measure all the ingredients accurately.
  - Double Boiling: Fill the small saucepan with water and heat it on low. Place the glass or stainless steel bowl in the saucepan, ensuring it doesn't touch the water.
  - Mix Ingredients: Add beeswax and coconut oil to the bowl. Stir gently until they melt together.
  - Incorporate Arrowroot Powder, Aloe Vera, and Vitamin E: Remove the bowl from heat once melted. Add arrowroot powder, aloe vera gel, and vitamin E oil. Mix thoroughly until a smooth, consistent mixture forms.
  - Transfer to Container: Carefully pour the clump-free mixture into the mascara tube or container. Allow it to cool and solidify before use.

Additional Tips

- *Texture Adjustments:* If the mascara seems too thick, add a touch more coconut oil. For a thinner consistency, increase the amount of aloe vera gel.
  - *Application:* Use a clean mascara wand. Wipe off excess product to avoid clumping during application.
  - *Storage:* Keep the mascara in a cool, dry place away from direct sunlight.

Caution

- ALWAYS CONDUCT A patch test before applying any homemade cosmetics around the eyes to check for allergic reactions.

Commercial Version

FOR COMMERCIAL PRODUCTION, consider adding natural preservatives to prolong shelf life. Enhance the formula with ingredients like jojoba oil for extra moisturization and to prevent clumps.

Ingredients for Commercial Version

- JOJOBA OIL (1/2 teaspoon)
  - Natural Preservative (As per manufacturer's guidelines)

Shelf Life & Packaging Tips

THE HOMEMADE CLUMP-free mascara, if stored properly, can last for around 3-6 months. With added natural preservatives for commercial use, it might have a shelf life of approximately 6-12 months. Dark-colored, airtight containers are recommended for preservation and to protect the mascara from light exposure.

Unique Selling Proposition (USP)

HIGHLIGHT THE MASCARA'S clump-free formula, emphasizing its organic ingredients that prevent clumping while nourishing lashes. Emphasize that this mascara provides a smooth, flawless application without the hassle of clumps.

Ingredients

1. Beeswax (1/2 teaspoon)

Beeswax provides structure and helps the lipstick maintain its shape. It also aids in creating a smooth texture for application.

2. Shea Butter (1 teaspoon)

SHEA BUTTER MOISTURIZES and nourishes the lips, preventing dryness and providing a creamy consistency to the lipstick.

3. Alkanet Root Powder (1/4 teaspoon)

ALKANET ROOT POWDER is a natural pigment that gives a rich red color to the lipstick. It's organic and safe for use on the lips.

4. Jojoba Oil (1/2 teaspoon)

JOJOBA OIL CONDITIONS and softens the lips while contributing to the lipstick's smooth texture and glossy finish.

5. Vitamin E Oil (2-3 drops)

VITAMIN E OIL ACTS as a natural preservative, extending the lipstick's shelf life while providing additional nourishment for the lips.

Tools Required

- SMALL SAUCEPAN
  - Glass or stainless steel bowl
  - Spoon for mixing
  - Empty lipstick container or mold
  - Small funnel (optional)

Method

Homemade Version

- PREPARE INGREDIENTS: Measure out all the ingredients accurately.
- Double Boiling: Fill the small saucepan with water and heat it on low. Place the glass or stainless steel bowl in the saucepan, ensuring it doesn't touch the water.
- Melt Beeswax and Shea Butter: Add beeswax and shea butter to the bowl. Stir gently until they melt together.
- Incorporate Alkanet Root Powder, Jojoba Oil, and Vitamin E: Remove the bowl from heat once melted. Add alkanet root powder, jojoba oil, and vitamin E oil. Mix thoroughly until a smooth, consistent mixture forms.
- Transfer to Container: Carefully pour the lipstick mixture into the lipstick container or mold. Allow it to cool and solidify before use.

Additional Tips

- *Color Intensity:* Adjust the amount of alkanet root powder for a deeper or lighter shade of red.
- *Texture Adjustments:* Increase shea butter for a creamier texture or add a touch more jojoba oil for a glossier finish.
- *Storage:* Keep the lipstick in a cool, dry place away from direct sunlight.

Caution

- ALWAYS PERFORM A patch test before applying any homemade cosmetics on the lips to check for allergic reactions.

Commercial Version

FOR COMMERCIAL PRODUCTION, adding natural preservatives might be necessary to extend shelf life. Also, consider enhancing the formula with additional ingredients like cocoa butter for added moisture and a smoother texture.

Ingredients for Commercial Version

- COCOA BUTTER (1 teaspoon)
  - Natural Preservative (As per manufacturer's guidelines)

Shelf Life & Packaging Tips

THE HOMEMADE RED LIPSTICK, if stored properly, can last for around 3-6 months. With added natural preservatives for commercial use, it might have a shelf life of approximately 6-12 months. Opt for lipstick tubes or containers that can be sealed airtight to preserve the lipstick.

Unique Selling Proposition (USP)

HIGHLIGHT THE LIPSTICK'S vibrant red color, organic ingredients, and moisturizing properties. Emphasize that this lipstick offers a natural and nourishing alternative to conventional lipsticks while providing a stunning red hue.

Ingredients

1. Beetroot Powder (1 tablespoon)

Beetroot powder provides the natural color pigment for the lip stain. It's organic, safe for use on the lips, and gives a lovely red hue.

2. Shea Butter (1 teaspoon)

SHEA BUTTER MOISTURIZES and nourishes the lips, preventing dryness and ensuring a smooth application of the lip stain.

3. Coconut Oil (1 teaspoon)

COCONUT OIL HYDRATES the lips and helps in achieving a creamy texture for the lip stain. It also aids in the application process.

4. Jojoba Oil (1/2 teaspoon)

JOJOBA OIL SOFTENS and conditions the lips, contributing to the smoothness of the lip stain and providing additional moisture.

5. Vitamin E Oil (2-3 drops)

VITAMIN E OIL ACTS as a natural preservative, extending the lip stain's shelf life while offering nourishment for the lips.

Tools Required

- SMALL SAUCEPAN
  - Glass or stainless steel bowl
  - Spoon for mixing
  - Empty lip balm or small jar/container
  - Small funnel (optional)

Method

Homemade Version

- PREPARE INGREDIENTS: Measure all the ingredients accurately.
  - Double Boiling: Fill the small saucepan with water and heat it on low. Place the glass or stainless steel bowl in the saucepan, ensuring it doesn't touch the water.
  - Mix Ingredients: Add shea butter and coconut oil to the bowl. Stir gently until they melt together.
  - Incorporate Beetroot Powder, Jojoba Oil, and Vitamin E: Remove the bowl from heat once melted. Add beetroot powder, jojoba oil, and vitamin E oil. Mix thoroughly until a smooth, consistent mixture forms.
  - Transfer to Container: Carefully pour the lip stain mixture into the lip balm container or small jar. Allow it to cool and solidify before use.

Additional Tips

- *Color Intensity:* Adjust the amount of beetroot powder for a lighter or deeper shade of red.
  - *Texture Adjustments:* Increase shea butter for a creamier texture or add more coconut oil for a glossier finish.
  - *Storage:* Keep the lip stain in a cool, dry place away from direct sunlight.

Caution

- ALWAYS PERFORM A patch test before applying any homemade cosmetics on the lips to check for allergic reactions.

Commercial Version

FOR COMMERCIAL PRODUCTION, adding natural preservatives might be necessary to extend shelf life. Consider enhancing the formula with additional ingredients like cocoa butter for extra moisture and a smoother texture.

Ingredients for Commercial Version

- COCOA BUTTER (1 teaspoon)
  - Natural Preservative (As per manufacturer's guidelines)

Shelf Life & Packaging Tips

THE HOMEMADE BEETROOT lip stain, if stored properly, can last for around 3-6 months. With added natural preservatives for commercial use, it might have a shelf life of approximately 6-12 months. Choose airtight containers for preservation and label them with ingredients and expiration dates.

Unique Selling Proposition (USP)

HIGHLIGHT THE LIP STAIN'S natural red color derived from organic beetroot powder. Emphasize its nourishing properties with organic ingredients, offering a chemical-free option for beautifully tinted lips. This lip stain provides a safe and natural alternative to conventional lip stains.

Organic Cocoa Butter Lip Balm

Ingredients

1. Cocoa Butter (2 tablespoons)

Cocoa butter deeply moisturizes and nourishes the lips, providing a protective layer against dryness and chapping. It helps in creating a smooth and soft texture for the lip balm.

2. Beeswax (1 tablespoon)

BEESWAX ACTS AS A NATURAL thickener and emulsifier in the lip balm, providing structure and helping it to solidify. It also offers a protective barrier for the lips.

3. Coconut Oil (1 tablespoon)

COCONUT OIL HYDRATES and conditions the lips, keeping them supple and preventing moisture loss. It contributes to the lip balm's creamy texture.

4. Vitamin E Oil (1 teaspoon)

VITAMIN E OIL ACTS as a natural preservative, extending the lip balm's shelf life while offering additional nourishment and antioxidants for the lips.

Tools Required

- SMALL SAUCEPAN
  - Glass or stainless steel bowl
  - Spoon for mixing
  - Empty lip balm containers or tubes
  - Small funnel (optional)

Method

Homemade Version

- PREPARE INGREDIENTS: Measure all the ingredients accurately.
- Double Boiling: Fill the small saucepan with water and heat it on low. Place the glass or stainless steel bowl in the saucepan, ensuring it doesn't touch the water.
- Melt Cocoa Butter, Beeswax, and Coconut Oil: Add cocoa butter, beeswax, and coconut oil to the bowl. Stir gently until they melt and combine.
- Incorporate Vitamin E Oil: Remove the bowl from heat once melted. Add vitamin E oil to the mixture and stir thoroughly.
- Pour into Containers: Carefully pour the liquid lip balm into the empty lip balm containers or tubes using a small funnel if needed. Allow it to cool and solidify before use.

Additional Tips

- *Scent or Flavor:* You can add a few drops of organic essential oils like peppermint or vanilla for a pleasant scent or flavor.
- *Texture Adjustments:* For a softer balm, increase the proportion of cocoa butter. To make it smoother, add more coconut oil.

Caution

- AVOID CONTACT WITH eyes. Perform a patch test before applying the lip balm to the lips to check for allergic reactions.

Commercial Version

FOR COMMERCIAL PRODUCTION, ensuring consistency and scalability is essential. Adding natural preservatives might be necessary to extend shelf life. You can also consider incorporating additional ingredients like shea butter for added moisturization and various organic essential oils for fragrance variations.

Ingredients for Commercial Version

- SHEA BUTTER (1 TABLESPOON)
  - Organic Essential Oils (As desired for scent)

Shelf Life & Packaging Tips

THE HOMEMADE COCOA butter lip balm, if stored properly, can last for around 6-12 months. With added natural preservatives for commercial use, it might have a shelf life of approximately 12-24 months. Use labeled, airtight containers or tubes for packaging to ensure hygiene and preservation.

Unique Selling Proposition (USP)

HIGHLIGHT THE LIP BALM'S organic cocoa butter content, which deeply nourishes and protects the lips. Emphasize its natural ingredients and moisturizing properties, providing long-lasting hydration and care for dry and chapped lips. This lip balm offers an organic solution for healthy and soft lips.

Organic Raspberry Seed Oil Tinted Lip Balm

Ingredients

1. Raspberry Seed Oil (2 tablespoons)

Raspberry seed oil is rich in antioxidants and essential fatty acids. It helps moisturize, soften, and protect the lips while providing a natural tint.

2. Beeswax (1 tablespoon)

BEESWAX ACTS AS A NATURAL thickener and emollient in the lip balm, providing structure and protecting the lips from external elements.

3. Shea Butter (1 tablespoon)

SHEA BUTTER DEEPLY nourishes and moisturizes the lips, aiding in softening and providing a creamy texture to the lip balm.

4. Coconut Oil (1 tablespoon)

COCONUT OIL HYDRATES and conditions the lips, keeping them smooth and preventing moisture loss. It contributes to the lip balm's softness.

5. Natural Red Pigment (Optional for additional tint)

NATURAL RED PIGMENT like beetroot powder or alkanet root powder can be added in small quantities to enhance the tint of the lip balm.

Tools Required

- SMALL SAUCEPAN
  - Glass or stainless steel bowl
  - Spoon for mixing
  - Empty lip balm containers or tubes
  - Small funnel (optional)

Method

Homemade Version

● PREPARE INGREDIENTS: Measure all the ingredients accurately.

● Double Boiling: Fill the small saucepan with water and heat it on low. Place the glass or stainless steel bowl in the saucepan, ensuring it doesn't touch the water.

● Melt Raspberry Seed Oil, Beeswax, Shea Butter, and Coconut Oil: Add raspberry seed oil, beeswax, shea butter, and coconut oil to the bowl. Stir gently until they melt and blend together.

● Optional: Add Natural Red Pigment: If using natural red pigment for additional tint, add it slowly and mix until desired color is achieved.

● Pour into Containers: Carefully pour the liquid lip balm into the empty lip balm containers or tubes using a small funnel if needed. Allow it to cool and solidify before use.

Additional Tips

● *Tint Intensity:* Adjust the amount of natural red pigment for a lighter or deeper tint.

● *Texture Adjustments:* Increase shea butter for a creamier texture or add more raspberry seed oil for extra hydration.

Caution

● PERFORM A PATCH test before applying any homemade cosmetics on the lips to check for allergic reactions.

Commercial Version

FOR COMMERCIAL PRODUCTION, maintaining consistency and scaling the recipe is important. Adding natural preservatives might be necessary to extend shelf life. You can also consider adding essential oils for fragrance variations or additional moisturizing agents like cocoa butter.

Ingredients for Commercial Version

- NATURAL PRESERVATIVE (As per manufacturer's guidelines)
  - Essential Oils (As desired for scent)

Shelf Life & Packaging Tips

THE HOMEMADE RASPBERRY seed oil tinted lip balm, if stored properly, can last for around 6-12 months. With added natural preservatives for commercial use, it might have a shelf life of approximately 12-24 months. Use labeled, airtight containers or tubes for packaging to ensure hygiene and preservation.

Unique Selling Proposition (USP)

HIGHLIGHT THE LIP BALM'S organic raspberry seed oil content, which provides both moisture and a natural tint. Emphasize its natural ingredients and the beautiful color it offers, catering to those seeking a tinted lip balm with organic components. This lip balm stands out for its hydrating properties and subtle tint.

Ingredients

1. Beetroot Powder (1 tablespoon)

Beetroot powder provides a natural red pigment for the lipstick. It's organic and safe, offering a vibrant red color without any synthetic dyes.

2. Cocoa Butter (2 tablespoons)

COCOA BUTTER DEEPLY moisturizes the lips and helps in creating a smooth texture for the lipstick. It ensures the lipstick glides on easily and stays hydrated.

3. Coconut Oil (1 tablespoon)

COCONUT OIL HYDRATES and nourishes the lips, preventing dryness and providing a glossy finish to the lipstick.

4. Almond Oil (1/2 tablespoon)

ALMOND OIL SOFTENS and conditions the lips while adding a silky texture to the lipstick.

5. Beeswax (1 tablespoon)

BEESWAX ACTS AS A NATURAL thickener and emollient, providing structure to the lipstick and aiding in its longevity.

Tools Required

- SMALL SAUCEPAN
  - Glass or stainless steel bowl
  - Spoon for mixing
  - Empty lipstick containers or molds
  - Small funnel (optional)

Method

Homemade Version

- PREPARE INGREDIENTS: Measure all the ingredients accurately.
- Double Boiling: Fill the small saucepan with water and heat it on low. Place the glass or stainless steel bowl in the saucepan, ensuring it doesn't touch the water.
- Melt Cocoa Butter, Coconut Oil, Almond Oil, and Beeswax: Add cocoa butter, coconut oil, almond oil, and beeswax to the bowl. Stir gently until they melt and blend together.
- Incorporate Beetroot Powder: Remove the bowl from heat once melted. Add beetroot powder gradually while stirring continuously until the desired red hue is achieved.
- Pour into Containers: Carefully pour the liquid lipstick into the empty lipstick containers or molds using a small funnel if needed. Allow it to cool and solidify before use.

Additional Tips

- *Color Intensity:* Adjust the amount of beetroot powder for a deeper or lighter red shade.
- *Texture Adjustments:* Increase cocoa butter for a creamier texture or add more coconut oil for a glossier finish.

Caution

- ALWAYS PERFORM A patch test before applying any homemade cosmetics on the lips to check for allergic reactions.

Commercial Version

FOR COMMERCIAL PRODUCTION, maintaining consistency and scalability is essential. Adding natural preservatives might be necessary to extend shelf life. Also, consider enhancing the formula with additional ingredients like vitamin E oil for its antioxidant properties.

Ingredients for Commercial Version

- VITAMIN E OIL (1 teaspoon)
  - Natural Preservative (As per manufacturer's guidelines)

Shelf Life & Packaging Tips

THE HOMEMADE RED VELVET lipstick, if stored properly, can last for around 6-12 months. With added natural preservatives for commercial use, it might have a shelf life of approximately 12-24 months. Use labeled, airtight lipstick containers for packaging to ensure hygiene and preservation.

Unique Selling Proposition (USP)

HIGHLIGHT THE LIPSTICK'S organic nature and its beautiful red hue derived from natural beetroot powder. Emphasize its moisturizing properties with organic ingredients, offering a chemical-free option for a vibrant and hydrating red lipstick. This lipstick stands out for its natural color and nourishing qualities.

Ingredients

1. Rose Petal Infused Oil (2 tablespoons)

Rose petal infused oil is rich in antioxidants and vitamins, soothing and hydrating the lips while providing a delicate rose scent.

2. Beeswax (1 tablespoon)

BEESWAX ACTS AS A NATURAL thickener and emollient, offering structure to the lipstick and aiding in its longevity.

3. Honey (1 tablespoon)

HONEY IS A NATURAL humectant, locking in moisture and keeping the lips soft and supple.

4. Alkanet Root Powder (1/2 teaspoon - Optional)

ALKANET ROOT POWDER adds a subtle reddish tint to the lipstick, enhancing its color naturally.

Tools Required

- SMALL SAUCEPAN
  - Glass or stainless steel bowl
  - Spoon for mixing
  - Empty lipstick containers or molds
  - Small funnel (optional)

Method

Homemade Version

- PREPARE INGREDIENTS: Measure all the ingredients accurately.

● Double Boiling: Fill the small saucepan with water and heat it on low. Place the glass or stainless steel bowl in the saucepan, ensuring it doesn't touch the water.

● Melt Rose Petal Infused Oil and Beeswax: Add rose petal infused oil and beeswax to the bowl. Stir gently until they melt and blend together.

● Incorporate Honey: Remove the bowl from heat once melted. Add honey and mix thoroughly.

● Optional: Add Alkanet Root Powder: If desired, gradually add alkanet root powder while stirring continuously until the desired tint is achieved.

● Pour into Containers: Carefully pour the liquid lipstick into the empty lipstick containers or molds using a small funnel if needed. Allow it to cool and solidify before use.

Additional Tips

● *Texture Adjustments:* Increase beeswax for a firmer texture or add more rose petal infused oil for a softer, glossier finish.

● *Fragrance Variation:* Incorporate a few drops of organic essential oils like rose or lavender for added fragrance.

Caution

● ALWAYS PERFORM A patch test before applying any homemade cosmetics on the lips to check for allergic reactions.

Commercial Version

FOR COMMERCIAL PRODUCTION, maintaining consistency and scalability is crucial. Adding natural preservatives might be necessary to extend shelf life. You can also consider adding vitamin E oil for additional nourishment and a longer-lasting formula.

Ingredients for Commercial Version

● VITAMIN E OIL (1 teaspoon)
  ● Natural Preservative (As per manufacturer's guidelines)

Shelf Life & Packaging Tips

THE HOMEMADE HONEYED rose lipstick, if stored properly, can last for around 6-12 months. With added natural preservatives for commercial use, it might have a shelf life of approximately 12-24 months. Use labeled, airtight lipstick containers for packaging to ensure hygiene and preservation.

Unique Selling Proposition (USP)

HIGHLIGHT THE LIPSTICK'S organic ingredients, especially the soothing properties of rose petal infused oil and honey. Emphasize its natural color enhancement from alkanet root powder and its hydrating effects for soft and scented lips. This lipstick stands out for its natural fragrance and moisturizing qualities.

Ingredients

1. Cocoa Butter (2 tablespoons)

Cocoa butter deeply moisturizes and nourishes the lips, leaving them soft and supple. It also provides a solid base for the lip balm.

2. Coconut Oil (1 tablespoon)

COCONUT OIL HYDRATES and conditions the lips, preventing moisture loss and ensuring they stay smooth.

3. Beeswax (1 tablespoon)

BEESWAX ACTS AS A NATURAL thickener and helps in solidifying the lip balm, providing structure and long-lasting hydration.

4. Peppermint Essential Oil (10-15 drops)

PEPPERMINT ESSENTIAL oil offers a refreshing and cooling sensation to the lips, along with a pleasant minty fragrance.

5. Vitamin E Oil (1/2 teaspoon)

VITAMIN E OIL IS RICH in antioxidants and helps in rejuvenating and protecting the delicate skin of the lips.

Tools Required

- SMALL SAUCEPAN
  - Glass or stainless steel bowl
  - Spoon for mixing
  - Empty lip balm containers or tubes
  - Small funnel (optional)

Method

Homemade Version

- PREPARE INGREDIENTS: Measure all the ingredients accurately.
- Double Boiling: Fill the small saucepan with water and heat it on low. Place the glass or stainless steel bowl in the saucepan, ensuring it doesn't touch the water.
- Melt Cocoa Butter, Coconut Oil, and Beeswax: Add cocoa butter, coconut oil, and beeswax to the bowl. Stir gently until they melt and blend together.
- Incorporate Peppermint Essential Oil and Vitamin E Oil: Remove the bowl from heat once melted. Add peppermint essential oil and vitamin E oil. Mix thoroughly.
- Pour into Containers: Carefully pour the liquid lip balm into the empty lip balm containers or tubes using a small funnel if needed. Allow it to cool and solidify before use.

Additional Tips

- *Adjusting Minty Flavor:* Increase or decrease the amount of peppermint essential oil for a stronger or milder minty sensation.
- *Texture Adjustments:* Increase beeswax for a firmer lip balm or add more coconut oil for a softer, glossy finish.

Caution

- PERFORM A PATCH test before applying any homemade cosmetics on the lips to check for allergic reactions, especially with essential oils.

Commercial Version

FOR COMMERCIAL PRODUCTION, maintaining consistency and scalability is vital. Adding natural preservatives might be necessary to extend shelf life. You can consider using organic peppermint leaves or natural flavor oils for a variation in the minty flavor.

Ingredients for Commercial Version

- NATURAL PRESERVATIVE (As per manufacturer's guidelines)
  - Organic Peppermint Leaves or Natural Flavor Oils (For variation)

Shelf Life & Packaging Tips

THE HOMEMADE MINTY cocoa lip balm, if stored properly, can last for around 6-12 months. With added natural preservatives for commercial use, it might have a shelf life of approximately 12-24 months. Use labeled, airtight lip balm containers for packaging to ensure hygiene and preservation.

Unique Selling Proposition (USP)

HIGHLIGHT THE LIP BALM'S organic ingredients, especially the soothing effects of cocoa butter and the refreshing minty sensation from peppermint essential oil. Emphasize its natural flavor and moisturizing properties, making it a cooling treat for the lips. This lip balm stands out for its minty freshness and organic goodness.

Ingredients

1. Beetroot Powder (1 tablespoon)

Beetroot powder provides a natural reddish pigment for the lipstick. It's organic and offers a vibrant color without any synthetic dyes.

2. Alkanet Root Powder (1/2 teaspoon - Optional)

ALKANET ROOT POWDER adds a deeper red or berry-like tint to the lipstick, enhancing its color naturally.

3. Coconut Oil (2 tablespoons)

COCONUT OIL MOISTURIZES and nourishes the lips, keeping them hydrated and soft.

4. Beeswax (1 tablespoon)

BEESWAX ACTS AS A NATURAL thickener, providing structure to the lipstick and aiding in its longevity.

5. Shea Butter (1 tablespoon)

SHEA BUTTER SOOTHES and protects the lips, locking in moisture and preventing dryness.

Tools Required

- SMALL SAUCEPAN
  - Glass or stainless steel bowl
  - Spoon for mixing
  - Empty lipstick containers or molds
  - Small funnel (optional)

Method

Homemade Version

- PREPARE INGREDIENTS: Measure all the ingredients accurately.
- Double Boiling: Fill the small saucepan with water and heat it on low. Place the glass or stainless steel bowl in the saucepan, ensuring it doesn't touch the water.
- Melt Coconut Oil, Beeswax, and Shea Butter: Add coconut oil, beeswax, and shea butter to the bowl. Stir gently until they melt and blend together.
- Incorporate Beetroot Powder and Alkanet Root Powder: Remove the bowl from heat once melted. Add beetroot powder gradually while stirring continuously. Optionally, add alkanet root powder for a deeper hue.
- Pour into Containers: Carefully pour the liquid lipstick into the empty lipstick containers or molds using a small funnel if needed. Allow it to cool and solidify before use.

Additional Tips

- *Color Variation:* Adjust the amount of beetroot and alkanet root powder for a lighter or deeper berry shade.
- *Texture Enhancement:* Increase beeswax for a firmer texture or add more coconut oil for a glossier finish.

Caution

- ALWAYS PERFORM A patch test before applying any homemade cosmetics on the lips to check for allergic reactions.

Commercial Version

FOR COMMERCIAL PRODUCTION, maintaining consistency is essential. Natural preservatives might be needed to extend shelf life. Consider adding vitamin E oil for additional nourishment and antioxidants.

Ingredients for Commercial Version

- VITAMIN E OIL (1 teaspoon)
  - Natural Preservative (As per manufacturer's guidelines)

Shelf Life & Packaging Tips

THE HOMEMADE BERRY stain lipstick, if stored properly, can last for around 6-12 months. With added natural preservatives for commercial use, it might have a shelf life of approximately 12-24 months. Use labeled, airtight lipstick containers for packaging to ensure hygiene and preservation.

Unique Selling Proposition (USP)

EMPHASIZE THE LIPSTICK'S organic nature and the beautiful berry-like shade derived from natural beetroot and alkanet root powders. Highlight its nourishing properties with organic oils and butters, offering a chemical-free option for a vibrant berry lip stain. This lipstick stands out for its natural color and moisturizing benefits.

Organic Lavender Vanilla Lip Balm

Ingredients

1. Beeswax (1 tablespoon)

Beeswax acts as a natural emollient, providing a protective layer to the lips and locking in moisture.

2. Coconut Oil (2 tablespoons)

COCONUT OIL HYDRATES and nourishes the lips, preventing dryness and promoting softness.

3. Shea Butter (1 tablespoon)

SHEA BUTTER SOOTHES and conditions the lips, offering deep moisturization and a smooth texture.

4. Lavender Essential Oil (10-15 drops)

LAVENDER ESSENTIAL oil provides a calming and aromatic scent while possessing potential calming properties for the skin.

5. Vanilla Extract or Vanilla Essential Oil (1/2 teaspoon)

VANILLA EXTRACT OR essential oil adds a delightful fragrance and a hint of sweetness to the lip balm.

Tools Required

- SMALL SAUCEPAN
  - Glass or stainless steel bowl
  - Spoon for mixing
  - Empty lip balm containers or tubes
  - Small funnel (optional)

Method

Homemade Version

- PREPARE INGREDIENTS: Measure all the ingredients accurately.
  - Double Boiling: Fill the small saucepan with water and heat it on low. Place the glass or stainless steel bowl in the saucepan, ensuring it doesn't touch the water.
  - Melt Beeswax, Coconut Oil, and Shea Butter: Add beeswax, coconut oil, and shea butter to the bowl. Stir gently until they melt and blend together.
  - Incorporate Lavender Essential Oil and Vanilla: Remove the bowl from heat once melted. Add lavender essential oil and vanilla extract or essential oil. Mix thoroughly.
  - Pour into Containers: Carefully pour the liquid lip balm into the empty lip balm containers or tubes using a small funnel if needed. Allow it to cool and solidify before use.

Additional Tips

- *Scent Intensity:* Adjust the amount of lavender essential oil or vanilla to suit your preference for fragrance intensity.
  - *Texture Modification:* Increase beeswax for a firmer balm or add more coconut oil for a smoother, glossier finish.

Caution

- CONDUCT A PATCH test before applying any homemade cosmetics on the lips to check for allergic reactions, particularly with essential oils.

Commercial Version

FOR COMMERCIAL PRODUCTION, maintaining consistency and scent longevity is vital. Consider adding natural preservatives and antioxidants like vitamin E oil to prolong shelf life and enhance the lip balm's nourishing properties.

Ingredients for Commercial Version

- VITAMIN E OIL (1 teaspoon)
  - Natural Preservative (As per manufacturer's guidelines)

Shelf Life & Packaging Tips

THE HOMEMADE LAVENDER vanilla lip balm, when stored properly, can last for around 6-12 months. With added natural preservatives for commercial use, it might have a shelf life of approximately 12-24 months. Use labeled, airtight lip balm containers for packaging to ensure hygiene and preservation.

Unique Selling Proposition (USP)

HIGHLIGHT THE LIP BALM'S organic ingredients, the soothing aroma of lavender, and the sweet, comforting scent of vanilla. Emphasize its natural fragrance and moisturizing effects, offering a calming and hydrating experience for the lips. This lip balm stands out for its organic essence and aromatic blend.

Ingredients

1. Shea Butter (1 tablespoon)

Shea butter provides moisture and nourishment to the lips, preventing dryness and maintaining softness.

2. Beeswax (1 tablespoon)

BEESWAX ACTS AS A NATURAL thickening agent, offering structure and texture to the lipstick while protecting the lips.

3. Jojoba Oil (1 tablespoon)

JOJOBA OIL CONDITIONS the lips, keeping them hydrated and aiding in a smooth application.

4. Arrowroot Powder (1 teaspoon)

ARROWROOT POWDER HELPS achieve the matte texture in the lipstick without the use of synthetic ingredients.

5. Natural Clay (1/2 teaspoon)

NATURAL CLAY, LIKE bentonite or kaolin, contributes to the matte finish and helps balance the lipstick's consistency.

Tools Required

- SMALL SAUCEPAN
  - Glass or stainless steel bowl
  - Spoon for mixing
  - Empty lipstick containers or molds
  - Small funnel (optional)

Method

Homemade Version

- PREPARE INGREDIENTS: Measure all the ingredients accurately.
  - Double Boiling: Fill the small saucepan with water and heat it on low. Place the glass or stainless steel bowl in the saucepan, ensuring it doesn't touch the water.
  - Melt Shea Butter and Beeswax: Add shea butter and beeswax to the bowl. Stir gently until they melt and blend together.
  - Incorporate Jojoba Oil, Arrowroot Powder, and Natural Clay: Remove the bowl from heat once melted. Add jojoba oil, arrowroot powder, and natural clay. Mix thoroughly until a consistent texture is achieved.
  - Pour into Containers: Carefully pour the lipstick mixture into the empty lipstick containers or molds using a small funnel if needed. Allow it to cool and solidify before use.

Additional Tips

- *Color Enhancement:* Incorporate natural mica powder or cocoa powder for a subtle tint.
  - *Matte Texture Variation:* Adjust the amount of arrowroot powder or natural clay to achieve the desired matte effect.

Caution

- PERFORM A PATCH test before applying any homemade cosmetics on the lips to check for allergic reactions.

Commercial Version

FOR COMMERCIAL PRODUCTION, maintaining consistency and color stability is essential. Adding natural preservatives might extend shelf life and ensure product safety.

Ingredients for Commercial Version

- VITAMIN E OIL (1 teaspoon)
  - Natural Preservative (As per manufacturer's guidelines)

Shelf Life & Packaging Tips

THE HOMEMADE NUDE MATTE lipstick, if stored properly, can last for around 6-12 months. With added natural preservatives for commercial use, it might have a shelf life of approximately 12-24 months. Use labeled, airtight lipstick containers for packaging to ensure hygiene and preservation.

Unique Selling Proposition (USP)

HIGHLIGHT THE LIPSTICK'S organic composition, offering a nude shade with a matte finish without synthetic additives. Emphasize its hydrating properties and natural matte look, providing a chemical-free option for a sophisticated, natural lip color. This lipstick stands out for its organic essence and subtle, elegant finish.

Organic Citrus Burst Lip Balm

Ingredients

1. Beeswax (1 tablespoon)

Beeswax acts as a natural emollient, providing a protective layer to the lips and sealing in moisture.

2. Coconut Oil (2 tablespoons)

COCONUT OIL HYDRATES and nourishes the lips, preventing dryness and offering a smooth texture.

3. Shea Butter (1 tablespoon)

SHEA BUTTER SOOTHES and conditions the lips, ensuring deep moisturization and softness.

4. Sweet Almond Oil (1 tablespoon)

SWEET ALMOND OIL HELPS to rejuvenate and revitalize the lips, keeping them supple and healthy.

5. Citrus Essential Oil Blend (10-15 drops)

CITRUS ESSENTIAL OILS, like orange, lemon, or grapefruit, provide a refreshing burst of fragrance and potential uplifting properties.

Tools Required

- SMALL SAUCEPAN
  - Glass or stainless steel bowl
  - Spoon for mixing
  - Empty lip balm containers or tubes
  - Small funnel (optional)

Method

Homemade Version

- PREPARE INGREDIENTS: Measure all the ingredients accurately.
  - Double Boiling: Fill the small saucepan with water and heat it on low. Place the glass or stainless steel bowl in the saucepan, ensuring it doesn't touch the water.
  - Melt Beeswax, Coconut Oil, and Shea Butter: Add beeswax, coconut oil, and shea butter to the bowl. Stir gently until they melt and blend together.
  - Incorporate Sweet Almond Oil and Citrus Essential Oil: Remove the bowl from heat once melted. Add sweet almond oil and the citrus essential oil blend. Mix thoroughly.
  - Pour into Containers: Carefully pour the liquid lip balm into the empty lip balm containers or tubes using a small funnel if needed. Allow it to cool and solidify before use.

Additional Tips

- *Scent Combination:* Experiment with different ratios of citrus essential oils for your preferred fragrance balance.
  - *Texture Adjustment:* Increase beeswax for a firmer balm or add more coconut oil for a softer, glossier finish.

Caution

- ALWAYS PATCH TEST homemade cosmetics on a small area of the skin to check for potential allergic reactions, especially with essential oils.

Commercial Version

TO CREATE A COMMERCIAL version, consider incorporating natural preservatives and antioxidants like vitamin E oil to prolong shelf life and maintain product integrity.

Ingredients for Commercial Version

- VITAMIN E OIL (1 teaspoon)
  - Natural Preservative (As per manufacturer's guidelines)

Shelf Life & Packaging Tips

THE HOMEMADE CITRUS burst lip balm, when stored properly, can last for around 6-12 months. With added natural preservatives for commercial use, it might have a shelf life of approximately 12-24 months. Use labeled, airtight lip balm containers for packaging to ensure hygiene and preservation.

Unique Selling Proposition (USP)

HIGHLIGHT THE LIP BALM'S organic components, offering a refreshing burst of citrus fragrance while providing deep moisturization. Emphasize its natural essence and the uplifting feel it provides, offering a revitalizing experience for the lips. This lip balm stands out for its organic essence and invigorating citrus burst.

Ingredients

1. Beeswax (1 tablespoon)

Beeswax forms a protective barrier on the lips, locking in moisture and preventing dryness.

2. Coconut Oil (2 tablespoons)

COCONUT OIL HYDRATES and nourishes the lips deeply, leaving them soft and supple.

3. Shea Butter (1 tablespoon)

SHEA BUTTER SOOTHES and conditions the lips, promoting smoothness and elasticity.

4. Sweet Almond Oil (1 tablespoon)

SWEET ALMOND OIL REJUVENATES and revitalizes the lips, helping maintain their health and moisture.

5. Lime Essential Oil (10-15 drops)

LIME ESSENTIAL OIL offers a refreshing citrus scent and potentially uplifting properties.

Tools Required

- SMALL SAUCEPAN
  - Glass or stainless steel bowl
  - Spoon for mixing
  - Empty lip balm containers or tubes
  - Small funnel (optional)

Method

Homemade Version

- PREPARE INGREDIENTS: Measure all the organic ingredients accurately.
  - Double Boiling: Fill the small saucepan with water and heat it on low. Place the glass or stainless steel bowl in the saucepan, ensuring it doesn't touch the water.
  - Melt Beeswax, Coconut Oil, and Shea Butter: Add beeswax, coconut oil, and shea butter to the bowl. Stir gently until they melt and blend together.
  - Incorporate Sweet Almond Oil and Lime Essential Oil: Remove the bowl from heat once melted. Add sweet almond oil and the lime essential oil drops. Mix thoroughly.
  - Pour into Containers: Carefully pour the liquid lip balm into the empty lip balm containers or tubes using a small funnel if needed. Allow it to cool and solidify before use.

Additional Tips

- *Fragrance Balance:* Adjust the number of lime essential oil drops for your preferred level of citrus scent.
  - *Consistency Modification:* For a firmer balm, increase the amount of beeswax; for a softer texture, add more coconut oil.

Caution

- ALWAYS CONDUCT A patch test before applying homemade cosmetics to ensure there are no adverse reactions, particularly with essential oils.

Commercial Version

FOR A COMMERCIAL VERSION, consider adding natural preservatives such as vitamin E oil and an FDA-approved antimicrobial agent to extend shelf life and maintain quality.

Ingredients for Commercial Version

- VITAMIN E OIL (1 teaspoon)
  - FDA-Approved Antimicrobial Agent (As per regulations)

Shelf Life & Packaging Tips

THE HOMEMADE COCONUT lime lip balm, when stored properly, can last for around 6-12 months. Incorporating natural preservatives for commercial use might extend its shelf life to approximately 12-24 months. Use labeled, airtight lip balm containers for packaging to ensure hygiene and preservation.

Unique Selling Proposition (USP)

EMPHASIZE THE LIP BALM'S organic nature, combining the hydrating properties of coconut oil and shea butter with the invigorating essence of lime. Highlight its ability to provide intense hydration and a refreshing burst of citrus, leaving lips feeling rejuvenated and moisturized. This lip balm stands out for its organic components and revitalizing coconut-lime essence.

Ingredients

1. Beeswax (1 tablespoon)

Beeswax acts as a natural emulsifier and gives structure to the lipstick.

2. Shea Butter (1 tablespoon)

SHEA BUTTER PROVIDES moisture and helps the lipstick glide smoothly on the lips.

3. Coconut Oil (2 tablespoons)

COCONUT OIL MOISTURIZES and nourishes the lips, leaving them soft and hydrated.

4. Alkanet Root Powder (1 teaspoon)

ALKANET ROOT POWDER lends a natural coral hue to the lipstick, imparting a beautiful tint.

5. Red Mica Powder (1/2 teaspoon)

RED MICA POWDER ADDS a shimmering effect and enhances the color vibrancy.

6. Vitamin E Oil (few drops)

VITAMIN E OIL ACTS as a natural preservative and promotes lip health.

Tools Required

- SMALL SAUCEPAN
  - Heatproof glass or stainless steel bowl
  - Spoon for mixing
  - Lipstick molds or empty lipstick tubes

- Small funnel (optional)

Method

Homemade Version

- PREPARE INGREDIENTS: Gather all organic ingredients and measure them accurately.

- Creating Base: In a small saucepan, create a double boiler by filling it with water and placing the heatproof bowl on top. Melt beeswax, shea butter, and coconut oil in the bowl over low-medium heat, stirring gently until combined.

- Adding Colorants: Incorporate alkanet root powder and red mica powder into the melted mixture. Stir continuously until you achieve a smooth and evenly colored liquid.

- Infusion: Allow the mixture to infuse on low heat for 5-10 minutes to extract the color from alkanet root powder.

- Adding Vitamin E: Remove from heat and add a few drops of vitamin E oil. Mix thoroughly.

- Pouring into Molds: Carefully pour the liquid lipstick mixture into lipstick molds or tubes using a small funnel if necessary. Let it cool and solidify before use.

Additional Tips

- *Adjust Color Intensity:* Control the shade of coral by adding more or less alkanet root powder.

- *Experiment with Shimmer:* Alter the amount of red mica powder for a more or less shimmering effect.

Caution

- ALWAYS PERFORM A patch test to ensure there are no allergic reactions to any ingredients, especially natural colorants.

Commercial Version

FOR COMMERCIAL PRODUCTION, consider using cosmetic-grade pigments for color stability and longer shelf life.

Ingredients for Commercial Version

- COSMETIC-GRADE CORAL Pigment (As per manufacturer's recommendation)

Shelf Life & Packaging Tips

THE HOMEMADE CORAL reef lipstick, when stored properly, can last around 6-12 months. Commercial versions with additional preservatives may extend shelf life to approximately 12-24 months. Utilize labeled, airtight lipstick molds or tubes for hygienic and secure packaging.

Unique Selling Proposition (USP)

HIGHLIGHT THE LIPSTICK'S organic nature, combining the hydrating properties of coconut oil and shea butter with the vibrant, natural coral hue from alkanet root powder. Emphasize its ability to provide nourishment, color, and shimmer in a single application, distinguishing it as an organic, coral-inspired beauty choice.

Organic Peppermint Swirl Lip Balm

Ingredients

1. Beeswax (1 tablespoon)

Beeswax acts as a natural emollient, locking in moisture and providing structure to the lip balm.

2. Shea Butter (1 tablespoon)

SHEA BUTTER DEEPLY nourishes and hydrates the lips, promoting softness and suppleness.

3. Coconut Oil (2 tablespoons)

COCONUT OIL OFFERS intensive moisturization, keeping the lips smooth and preventing dryness.

4. Peppermint Essential Oil (10-15 drops)

PEPPERMINT OIL ADDS a refreshing scent and a mild cooling sensation to the lip balm.

5. Vitamin E Oil (few drops)

VITAMIN E OIL ACTS as a natural antioxidant, supporting lip health and preventing damage.

Tools Required

- SMALL SAUCEPAN
  - Heatproof glass or stainless steel bowl
  - Spoon for stirring
  - Lip balm containers or tubes
  - Small funnel (optional)

Method

Homemade Version

● GATHER INGREDIENTS: Assemble all organic ingredients needed for the lip balm recipe.

● Melt Ingredients: Create a double boiler by placing the heatproof bowl over a saucepan filled with water. Melt beeswax, shea butter, and coconut oil in the bowl over low heat, stirring gently until they combine.

● Add Peppermint Oil: Once melted, remove the mixture from heat and add peppermint essential oil and a few drops of vitamin E oil. Stir well to ensure even distribution.

● Pour into Containers: Carefully pour the liquid lip balm mixture into lip balm containers or tubes, using a small funnel if necessary. Allow it to cool and solidify before sealing the containers.

Additional Tips

● *Adjust Peppermint Intensity:* Control the strength of the peppermint scent by varying the amount of peppermint oil.

● *Test Before Use:* Always do a patch test on a small area to ensure no adverse reactions to the ingredients.

Caution

● BE CAUTIOUS WITH the amount of essential oil used, especially if applying to sensitive skin.

Commercial Version

FOR A COMMERCIAL VERSION, considering using higher-grade, certified organic ingredients and lab-tested peppermint oil.

Ingredients for Commercial Version

● CERTIFIED ORGANIC Peppermint Oil (As per regulatory guidelines)
● Certified Organic Beeswax

- Certified Organic Shea Butter
- Certified Organic Coconut Oil

Shelf Life & Packaging Tips

HOMEMADE PEPPERMINT swirl lip balm can typically last around 6-12 months if stored in a cool, dry place. For commercial use, the addition of natural preservatives may extend the shelf life to 12-24 months. Ensure the lip balm containers are sanitized, airtight, and labeled properly for commercial packaging.

Unique Selling Proposition (USP)

HIGHLIGHT THE LIP BALM'S organic ingredients, focusing on the hydrating properties of coconut oil and shea butter blended with the refreshing sensation of peppermint essential oil. Emphasize its ability to provide long-lasting moisture and a delightful peppermint scent, making it a perfect everyday organic lip care choice.

Ingredients

1. Beeswax (1 tablespoon)

Beeswax helps give structure to the lipstick and provides a smooth texture for easy application.

2. Shea Butter (1 tablespoon)

SHEA BUTTER DEEPLY moisturizes and nourishes the lips, preventing dryness and flakiness.

3. Coconut Oil (2 tablespoons)

COCONUT OIL ACTS AS a base, contributing to the lipstick's creamy consistency and providing hydration.

4. Alkanet Root Powder (1 teaspoon)

ALKANET ROOT POWDER gives the lipstick its beautiful mauve hue, offering a natural and organic colorant.

5. Beetroot Powder (1/2 teaspoon)

BEETROOT POWDER ADDS depth and richness to the mauve shade, enhancing the color profile organically.

6. Vitamin E Oil (few drops)

VITAMIN E OIL ACTS as an antioxidant, supporting lip health and preventing damage.

Tools Required

- SMALL SAUCEPAN
  - Heatproof glass or stainless steel bowl

- Spoon for stirring
- Lipstick molds or empty lipstick tubes
- Small funnel (optional)

Method

Homemade Version

- COMBINE INGREDIENTS: In a heatproof bowl, melt beeswax, shea butter, and coconut oil over low heat using a double boiler setup.
- Add Colorants: Once melted, add alkanet root powder and beetroot powder, stirring continuously until the desired shade is achieved. Adjust the quantities for preferred color intensity.
- Incorporate Vitamin E: Remove the mixture from heat and add a few drops of vitamin E oil, blending it well into the lipstick mixture.
- Pour into Molds: Carefully pour the lipstick mixture into molds or lipstick tubes, using a small funnel if needed. Allow it to cool and solidify before sealing the containers.

Additional Tips

- *Color Intensity Adjustment:* Experiment with the quantity of alkanet root and beetroot powder to achieve the desired mauve shade.
- *Texture Modification:* Add more coconut oil for a creamier texture or increase beeswax for a firmer lipstick.

Caution

- PATCH TEST THE LIPSTICK on a small area of skin to ensure no allergic reactions to any of the ingredients.

Commercial Version

CONSIDER USING COSMETIC-grade, certified organic ingredients and undergo proper product testing and certification for commercial sale.

Ingredients for Commercial Version

- CERTIFIED ORGANIC Beeswax
  - Certified Organic Shea Butter
  - Certified Organic Coconut Oil
  - Certified Organic Alkanet Root Powder
  - Certified Organic Beetroot Powder

Shelf Life & Packaging Tips

HOMEMADE LIPSTICK TYPICALLY has a shelf life of 6-12 months when stored in a cool, dry place. For commercial use, incorporating natural preservatives can extend the shelf life to 12-24 months. Properly labeled and sealed lipstick tubes or packaging designed for commercial sale are essential.

Unique Selling Proposition (USP)

EMPHASIZE THE ORGANIC ingredients' benefits, highlighting the nourishing properties of shea butter and coconut oil blended with natural colorants like alkanet root and beetroot powder. Showcase the lipstick's mauve shade, offering a delightful and organic option for a beautiful lip color while maintaining lip health.

Ingredients

1. Beeswax (1 tablespoon)

Beeswax acts as a natural emollient, creating a protective barrier to retain moisture on the lips.

2. Shea Butter (1 tablespoon)

SHEA BUTTER DEEPLY moisturizes and softens the lips, promoting smoothness and preventing dryness.

3. Coconut Oil (2 tablespoons)

COCONUT OIL PROVIDES hydration and nourishment, keeping the lips supple and healthy.

4. Almond Oil (1 tablespoon)

ALMOND OIL IS RICH in vitamin E and works to soothe and condition the lips, aiding in healing and repair.

5. Honey (1 teaspoon)

HONEY OFFERS NATURAL antibacterial properties while adding a hint of sweetness to the balm.

Tools Required

- SMALL SAUCEPAN
  - Heatproof glass or stainless steel bowl
  - Spoon for stirring
  - Lip balm containers or tins
  - Small funnel (optional)

Method

Homemade Version

- MELT INGREDIENTS: In a heatproof bowl, combine beeswax, shea butter, coconut oil, and almond oil. Melt the mixture over low heat using a double boiler setup until fully liquefied.
  - Add Honey: Remove the bowl from heat and allow it to cool slightly. Stir in the honey gently until well incorporated into the mixture.
  - Pour into Containers: Carefully pour the lip balm mixture into lip balm containers or tins. Use a small funnel for precision if needed. Let it cool and solidify completely before sealing the containers.

Additional Tips

- *Adjusting Consistency:* Increase the amount of beeswax for a firmer balm or add more coconut oil for a softer texture.
  - *Scent Enhancement:* Consider adding a few drops of essential oil (like vanilla or lavender) for a fragrant touch.

Caution

PERFORM A PATCH TEST to check for any allergic reactions to the ingredients before applying the balm to your lips.

Commercial Version

FOR A COMMERCIAL VERSION, sourcing certified organic ingredients is crucial. Consider complying with cosmetic manufacturing standards and ensuring proper product testing.

Ingredients for Commercial Version

- CERTIFIED ORGANIC Beeswax
  - Certified Organic Shea Butter
  - Certified Organic Coconut Oil
  - Certified Organic Almond Oil

- Certified Organic Honey

Shelf Life & Packaging Tips

HOMEMADE LIP BALM TYPICALLY has a shelf life of 6-12 months when stored in a cool, dry place. To extend the shelf life for commercial purposes, incorporating natural preservatives and proper packaging techniques is recommended. Opt for airtight, labeled lip balm containers suitable for retail sale.

Unique Selling Proposition (USP)

HIGHLIGHT THE NATURAL moisturizing properties of shea butter, coconut oil, and almond oil, combined with the antibacterial benefits of organic honey, offering a luxurious lip balm experience. Emphasize the balm's organic nature and its ability to soothe, heal, and protect lips with a delightful hint of honey sweetness.

Ingredients

1. Shea Butter (1 tablespoon)

Shea butter deeply moisturizes and nourishes the lips, preventing dryness and flakiness.

2. Almond Oil (1 tablespoon)

ALMOND OIL SOFTENS and conditions the lips, providing a natural glow and suppleness.

3. Beeswax (1 tablespoon)

BEESWAX ACTS AS A NATURAL emollient, forming a protective layer on the lips to lock in moisture.

4. Peach Powder (1 teaspoon)

ORGANIC PEACH POWDER provides the desired peachy hue to the lipstick, adding a natural tint.

5. Vitamin E Oil (1 capsule)

VITAMIN E OIL PROMOTES lip health, acting as an antioxidant to prevent damage and maintain softness.

Tools Required

- SMALL SAUCEPAN
  - Heatproof glass or stainless steel bowl
  - Spoon for stirring
  - Lipstick molds or empty lipstick containers
  - Small funnel (optional)

Method

Homemade Version

● MELT INGREDIENTS: Combine shea butter, almond oil, and beeswax in a heatproof bowl. Melt the mixture over low heat using a double boiler setup until fully liquid.

● Add Peach Powder: Remove the bowl from heat and allow it to cool slightly. Mix in the organic peach powder until the color is evenly distributed throughout the mixture.

● Incorporate Vitamin E: Carefully pierce a vitamin E oil capsule and squeeze the contents into the bowl. Stir thoroughly to incorporate the oil.

● Pour into Containers: Using a small funnel if needed, pour the lipstick mixture into lipstick molds or empty lipstick containers. Let it cool and solidify completely before sealing the containers.

Additional Tips

● *Adjust Color Intensity:* Increase or decrease the amount of peach powder for a lighter or more intense hue.

● *Texture Modification:* Adjust the ratio of beeswax to achieve the desired consistency—more beeswax for a firmer lipstick and less for a softer texture.

Caution

ALWAYS PERFORM A PATCH test to check for any allergic reactions to the ingredients before applying the lipstick to your lips.

Commercial Version

FOR A COMMERCIAL VERSION, consider sourcing certified organic ingredients to align with cosmetic standards. Comply with relevant manufacturing regulations and conduct necessary product testing.

Ingredients for Commercial Version

- CERTIFIED ORGANIC Shea Butter
  - Certified Organic Almond Oil
  - Certified Organic Beeswax
  - Certified Organic Peach Powder
  - Vitamin E Oil (Ensure it meets commercial standards)

Shelf Life & Packaging Tips

HOMEMADE LIPSTICKS typically have a shelf life of 6-12 months when stored in a cool, dry place. To extend the shelf life for commercial purposes, consider incorporating natural preservatives and investing in professional-grade packaging suitable for retail sale.

Unique Selling Proposition (USP)

HIGHLIGHT THE ORGANIC ingredients' ability to moisturize, nourish, and color the lips naturally. Emphasize the creamy texture and the subtle, peachy tint that adds a touch of freshness to lips. Promote it as a natural, organic alternative for those seeking both color and lip care in one product.

Soothing Chamomile Lip Balm

Ingredients

1. Beeswax (2 tablespoons)

Beeswax forms a protective barrier on the lips, locking in moisture while providing a solid base for the lip balm.

2. Coconut Oil (3 tablespoons)

COCONUT OIL DEEPLY nourishes and hydrates the lips, aiding in softening and preventing chapping.

3. Shea Butter (2 tablespoons)

SHEA BUTTER IS RICH in vitamins and fatty acids, promoting smoothness and healing for dry or cracked lips.

4. Chamomile Infused Oil (2 tablespoons)

ORGANIC CHAMOMILE-INFUSED oil soothes and calms the lips, offering anti-inflammatory properties to reduce irritation.

5. Vitamin E Oil (1 teaspoon)

VITAMIN E OIL ACTS as a natural antioxidant, supporting the health of the lips and preventing damage.

Tools Required

- SMALL SAUCEPAN
  - Heatproof glass or stainless steel bowl
  - Spoon for stirring
  - Lip balm containers or tins
  - Small funnel (optional)

Method

Homemade Version

● PREPARE INFUSED Oil: Infuse dried chamomile flowers in a carrier oil (like olive oil) in advance. Strain the oil after 2-3 weeks for use.

● Melt Ingredients: In a heatproof bowl over a saucepan of simmering water, combine beeswax, coconut oil, shea butter, and chamomile-infused oil. Stir until melted.

● Incorporate Vitamin E: Remove the mixture from heat and add vitamin E oil. Stir to combine thoroughly.

● Pour into Containers: Carefully pour the liquid lip balm into lip balm containers or tins. Use a small funnel if needed. Let it cool and solidify completely before sealing.

Additional Tips

● *Adjust Chamomile Infusion:* For a stronger chamomile scent and properties, increase the amount of chamomile-infused oil.

● *Experiment with Texture:* Modify the beeswax amount to achieve a softer or firmer lip balm consistency.

Caution

BEFORE REGULAR USE, test a small amount of the balm on your skin to ensure no allergic reactions to any of the ingredients.

Commercial Version

TO PRODUCE THIS LIP balm for commercial purposes, source certified organic ingredients and adhere to manufacturing regulations. Explore natural preservatives for longer shelf life and consider professional-grade packaging suitable for retail.

Ingredients for Commercial Version

● CERTIFIED ORGANIC Beeswax

- Certified Organic Coconut Oil
- Certified Organic Shea Butter
- Certified Organic Chamomile Extract/Oil
- Vitamin E Oil (Ensure it meets commercial standards)

Shelf Life & Packaging Tips

HOMEMADE LIP BALMS typically last 6-12 months. For commercial use, consider incorporating natural preservatives for an extended shelf life and opt for appealing, eco-friendly packaging to attract customers.

Unique Selling Proposition (USP)

PROMOTE THE LIP BALM as a natural solution for soothing and calming dry, irritated lips. Highlight the organic ingredients' ability to provide deep hydration, while chamomile infusion adds a gentle and relaxing touch to the product.

Refreshing Eucalyptus Mint Lip Balm

Ingredients

1. Beeswax (2 tablespoons)

Beeswax acts as a natural emollient, creating a protective layer on the lips to retain moisture.

2. Coconut Oil (3 tablespoons)

COCONUT OIL DEEPLY hydrates and nourishes the lips, helping to prevent dryness and chapping.

3. Shea Butter (2 tablespoons)

SHEA BUTTER CONTAINS vitamins and fatty acids that promote softness and rejuvenation for the lips.

4. Eucalyptus Essential Oil (10 drops)

ORGANIC EUCALYPTUS oil offers a refreshing sensation and possesses antibacterial properties, ideal for soothing the lips.

5. Peppermint Essential Oil (10 drops)

PEPPERMINT OIL PROVIDES a cooling effect and helps to freshen and revitalize the lips.

Tools Required

- SMALL SAUCEPAN
  - Heatproof glass or stainless steel bowl
  - Spoon for stirring
  - Lip balm containers or tins
  - Small funnel (optional)

Method

Homemade Version

● MELT INGREDIENTS: In a heatproof bowl placed over a saucepan of simmering water, combine beeswax, coconut oil, and shea butter. Stir until melted.

● Add Essential Oils: Remove the mixture from heat and add eucalyptus and peppermint essential oils. Stir gently to ensure even distribution.

● Pour into Containers: Carefully pour the melted lip balm into lip balm containers or tins. Allow it to cool and solidify completely before sealing.

Additional Tips

● *Adjust Essential Oils:* Modify the amount of eucalyptus and peppermint oils based on your preference for fragrance and intensity.

● *Test for Sensitivity:* Prior to regular use, apply a small amount of the balm to the skin to ensure no allergic reactions to the ingredients.

Caution

BE CAUTIOUS WHEN USING essential oils directly on the skin. Always dilute them properly and avoid contact with eyes.

Commercial Version

FOR A COMMERCIAL VERSION, source certified organic ingredients and follow manufacturing regulations. Consider adding natural preservatives to extend shelf life and opt for professional-grade packaging suitable for retail.

Ingredients for Commercial Version

● CERTIFIED ORGANIC Beeswax
● Certified Organic Coconut Oil
● Certified Organic Shea Butter

- Organic Eucalyptus Essential Oil
- Organic Peppermint Essential Oil

Shelf Life & Packaging Tips

HOMEMADE LIP BALMS typically last 6-12 months. For commercial use, consider incorporating natural preservatives for a longer shelf life. Eye-catching, eco-friendly packaging can enhance product appeal.

Unique Selling Proposition (USP)

PROMOTE THE LIP BALM as a refreshing, organic solution for dry lips. Highlight the eucalyptus and peppermint combination for a cool, revitalizing experience, perfect for daily lip care.

Ingredients

1. Beeswax (2 tablespoons)

Beeswax acts as a natural emollient, forming a protective layer on the lips.

2. Coconut Oil (2 tablespoons)

ORGANIC COCONUT OIL deeply moisturizes the lips, preventing dryness.

3. Shea Butter (1 tablespoon)

SHEA BUTTER IS RICH in vitamins, promoting soft and supple lips.

4. Alkanet Root Powder (1/2 teaspoon)

ALKANET ROOT POWDER imparts a beautiful berry hue to the lipstick.

5. Raspberry Seed Oil (1 teaspoon)

RASPBERRY SEED OIL provides antioxidants and nutrients for lip nourishment.

6. Vitamin E Oil (1/2 teaspoon)

VITAMIN E OIL HELPS in moisturizing and provides anti-aging benefits for the lips.

Tools Required

- SMALL SAUCEPAN
  - Heatproof glass or stainless steel bowl
  - Spoon for stirring
  - Lipstick tubes or containers
  - Small funnel (optional)

Method

Homemade Version

● PREPARE OIL INFUSION: In a heatproof bowl, combine coconut oil, shea butter, and alkanet root powder. Place it over a saucepan of simmering water for 20 minutes. Remove and strain the infused oil.

● Combine Ingredients: In a clean bowl, mix the strained oil with beeswax, raspberry seed oil, and vitamin E oil. Heat the mixture until the beeswax melts completely.

● Pour into Containers: Once melted and well combined, carefully pour the mixture into lipstick tubes or containers. Allow it to cool and solidify before sealing.

Additional Tips

● *Color Intensity:* Adjust the amount of alkanet root powder for a lighter or more intense color.

● *Texture Enhancement:* Add more beeswax for a firmer lipstick or more coconut oil for a smoother texture.

Caution

BEFORE APPLICATION, test the lipstick on a small patch of skin to check for any allergic reactions.

Commercial Version

FOR A COMMERCIAL VERSION, source certified organic ingredients and adhere to manufacturing regulations. Consider adding natural preservatives to extend the shelf life and create a more stable product.

Ingredients for Commercial Version

● CERTIFIED ORGANIC Beeswax
● Certified Organic Coconut Oil
● Certified Organic Shea Butter

- Alkanet Root Extract (oil-soluble)
- Certified Organic Raspberry Seed Oil
- Natural Vitamin E Oil

Shelf Life & Packaging Tips

HOMEMADE LIPSTICKS typically last around 6 months to a year. Commercial versions might benefit from natural preservatives for a longer shelf life. Use sleek, eco-friendly packaging to enhance product appeal.

Unique Selling Proposition (USP)

EMPHASIZE THE ORGANIC ingredients and the nourishing properties of raspberry seed oil. Highlight the vibrant berry hue achieved naturally from alkanet root powder, offering a delightful berry sorbet color for the lips.

Ingredients

1. Beeswax (2 tablespoons)

Beeswax creates a protective barrier and seals in moisture for hydrated lips.

2. Coconut Oil (2 tablespoons)

ORGANIC COCONUT OIL deeply moisturizes and nourishes the lips.

3. Shea Butter (1 tablespoon)

SHEA BUTTER IS RICH in vitamins and antioxidants, promoting soft and smooth lips.

4. Lemon Essential Oil (10 drops)

LEMON ESSENTIAL OIL offers a refreshing scent and contributes to a rejuvenating effect on the lips.

5. Vitamin E Oil (1/2 teaspoon)

VITAMIN E OIL PROVIDES additional nourishment and helps maintain lip health.

Tools Required

- SMALL SAUCEPAN
  - Heatproof glass or stainless steel bowl
  - Spoon for stirring
  - Lip balm containers or tubes
  - Small funnel (optional)

Method

Homemade Version

- MELT INGREDIENTS: In a heatproof bowl, combine beeswax, coconut oil, and shea butter. Place the bowl over a saucepan with simmering water until everything melts together.
  - Add Essential Oil: Once melted, remove from heat and add lemon essential oil and vitamin E oil. Stir the mixture thoroughly.
  - Transfer to Containers: Carefully pour the mixture into lip balm containers or tubes. Let it cool and solidify before sealing.

Additional Tips

- *Adjusting Scent:* Vary the amount of lemon essential oil for a stronger or milder lemon scent.
  - *Texture Enhancement:* Add more beeswax for a firmer balm or more coconut oil for a smoother texture.

Caution

TEST THE LIP BALM ON a small area of skin to ensure no allergic reactions occur before widespread use.

Commercial Version

FOR A COMMERCIAL PRODUCT, source certified organic ingredients and adhere to safety and manufacturing regulations. Consider stability testing and add natural preservatives for an extended shelf life.

Ingredients for Commercial Version

- CERTIFIED ORGANIC Beeswax
  - Certified Organic Coconut Oil
  - Certified Organic Shea Butter
  - Lemon Essential Oil (Certified Organic)
  - Natural Vitamin E Oil

Shelf Life & Packaging Tips

HOMEMADE LIP BALMS typically last around 6 months to a year. To extend shelf life in a commercial version, consider adding natural preservatives. Opt for eco-friendly, compact packaging for easy use and portability.

Unique Selling Proposition (USP)

HIGHLIGHT THE ORGANIC ingredients and the invigorating lemon scent. Emphasize the moisturizing and revitalizing properties of the balm, offering a refreshing experience for the lips.

Homemade Natural Nail Polish (Various Colors)

Ingredients

1. Clear Nail Polish (1 bottle)

Clear nail polish forms the base for creating various colored nail polishes.

2. Natural Pigments

- *For Red/Pink:* Beetroot Powder (1 teaspoon)
  - *For Yellow/Orange:* Turmeric Powder (1 teaspoon)
  - *For Green:* Spirulina Powder (1 teaspoon)
  - *For Blue/Purple:* Butterfly Pea Flower Powder (1 teaspoon)
  - *For Brown:* Cocoa Powder (1 teaspoon)

3. Mixing Medium

- ETHYL ALCOHOL (1 tablespoon)
  - Clear Nail Polish Thinner (1 tablespoon)

Tools Required

- SMALL BOWLS OR CONTAINERS (for mixing colors)
  - Toothpicks or small stirring rods
  - Funnel (optional)
  - Small dropper or syringe (for precise mixing)

Method

Making Homemade Nail Polish

• PREPARE THE COLORS: In separate containers, mix each natural pigment with a few drops of ethyl alcohol to create a smooth paste for each color.

• Mix with Clear Polish: Add the desired amount of each pigment paste into the clear nail polish bottle using a small funnel or dropper. Use a toothpick to stir and blend the colors thoroughly.

• Adjust Consistency: If needed, add nail polish thinner drop by drop to achieve the desired consistency.

• Test & Refine: Apply a small amount on a nail to test the color. Adjust the color intensity by adding more pigment or clear polish accordingly.

Additional Tips

• *Layering Colors:* Experiment by layering colors to create unique shades.

• *Creating Pastels:* Dilute pigments with more clear polish for pastel hues.

• *Matte Finish:* Mix a small amount of cornstarch with clear polish for a matte effect.

Caution

ENSURE GOOD VENTILATION when using ethyl alcohol and work in a well-ventilated area.

Commercial Version

FOR COMMERCIAL PRODUCTION, ensure compliance with safety standards and regulations. Source certified organic pigments and adhere to proper manufacturing practices. Consider stability testing and add natural preservatives for longevity.

Ingredients for Commercial Version

- CERTIFIED ORGANIC Clear Nail Polish
  - Certified Organic Natural Pigments (in larger quantities)
  - Ethyl Alcohol (Certified Organic)
  - Clear Nail Polish Thinner (Certified Organic)

Shelf Life & Packaging Tips

HOMEMADE NAIL POLISH typically lasts up to a year. In a commercial setting, consider adding natural preservatives to extend the shelf life. Opt for eco-friendly packaging that highlights the organic and natural aspects of the product.

Unique Selling Proposition (USP)

EMPHASIZE THE NATURAL and organic pigments used, catering to individuals looking for non-toxic nail polish options. Highlight the versatility to create a wide array of colors using simple, organic ingredients.

Title: Silken Matte: Organic DIY Nail Polish for a Chic Finish

Ingredients:

● Organic Cornstarch (2 teaspoons): Adds thickness for a matte texture without harmful chemicals.

● Kaolin Clay (1 teaspoon): Provides a smooth finish and absorbs excess oil.

● Organic Pigment Powder (1/2 teaspoon): Adds color naturally without synthetic dyes.

● Clear Organic Nail Polish (2 tablespoons): Acts as a base for the matte polish.

● Essential Oil (4 drops): Optional for fragrance, choose organic options for a natural scent.

Why these ingredients?

● *Organic Cornstarch*: It thickens the polish, creating the desired matte effect without resorting to harmful substances.

● *Kaolin Clay*: This natural clay helps in achieving a smooth and matte finish while absorbing excess oil.

● *Organic Pigment Powder*: Adds color without synthetic dyes, keeping the recipe organic and safe.

● *Clear Organic Nail Polish*: Serves as the base for the matte polish, ensuring adhesion and longevity.

● *Essential Oil*: If used, adds a natural fragrance without synthetic additives.

Tools:

● SMALL MIXING BOWL
● Mixing Spoon or Stick
● Small Funnel
● Nail Polish Bottles or Containers

Method:

Homemade Version:

● PREPARATION: ENSURE the mixing bowl and spoon are clean and dry.

● Mixing: Combine the cornstarch, kaolin clay, and pigment powder in the bowl. Blend thoroughly.

● Add Base: Pour the clear organic nail polish into the dry mixture. Stir until fully combined and smooth.

● Scent (Optional): Add essential oil drops for fragrance, if desired. Mix well.

● Bottling: Use the funnel to pour the mixture into nail polish bottles or containers. Seal tightly.

Additional Tips:

● *Consistency Check*: Adjust cornstarch for a thicker texture or clear polish for a lighter matte effect.

● *Experimentation*: Try different pigment powders for various colors but ensure they are organic and safe.

● *Stirring*: Mix well to avoid clumps and achieve a uniform polish.

Caution:

● *Allergic Reactions*: Before use, test a small amount on a patch of skin to check for any allergic reactions to the ingredients.

Commercial Version:

Considerations:

● CREATING A COMMERCIAL version could be a great idea for a niche market seeking organic nail care.

● For commercial use, enhancing the formula for longevity and quality is vital.

● Increasing quantities would be necessary for mass production.

Additional Ingredients for Commercial Version:

● ORGANIC TAPIOCA Starch (1 teaspoon): Enhances consistency and shelf life.

● Natural Preservative (as recommended for cosmetics): Increases shelf life for retail purposes.

Why these additional ingredients?

● *Organic Tapioca Starch*: Improves consistency and aids in prolonging shelf life for commercial distribution.

● *Natural Preservative*: Crucial for retail sales, preventing bacterial growth and extending shelf life.

Shelf Life:

● HOMEMADE VERSION: Best used within a month for optimal quality.

● Commercial Version: With added preservatives, shelf life can extend to 6-12 months.

Packaging Tips:

● USE DARK-COLORED or opaque bottles to preserve the polish from light exposure.

● Include clear labeling emphasizing the organic, natural, and matte attributes.

Unique Selling Point (USP):

● PROMOTE THE POLISH as a unique, organic, and environmentally friendly option for those seeking a matte finish without harmful chemicals.

Clear Gloss: Organic DIY Glossy Nail Polish for a Stunning Shine

Ingredients:

- Clear Organic Nail Polish (3 tablespoons): Acts as the base for the glossy polish.
- Organic Jojoba Oil (1 teaspoon): Adds shine and promotes nail health.
- Organic Vitamin E Oil (1/2 teaspoon): Nourishes nails and enhances glossiness.
- Organic Lavender Essential Oil (4 drops): Optional for a natural fragrance.

Why these ingredients?

- *Clear Organic Nail Polish*: Provides the base for the glossy finish, ensuring adhesion and longevity.
- *Organic Jojoba Oil*: Adds shine to nails while providing moisture and promoting nail health.
- *Organic Vitamin E Oil*: Nourishes nails and cuticles, enhancing the glossiness of the polish.
- *Organic Lavender Essential Oil*: Optional for a pleasant natural fragrance.

Tools:

- SMALL MIXING BOWL
- Mixing Spoon or Stick
- Small Funnel
- Nail Polish Bottles or Containers

Method:

Homemade Version:

PREPARATION: ENSURE cleanliness of the mixing bowl and spoon.

Base Mix: Pour the clear organic nail polish into the mixing bowl.

Oil Addition: Add jojoba oil and vitamin E oil into the polish. Mix thoroughly.

Optional Fragrance: If desired, add drops of lavender essential oil. Stir well.

Bottling: Use a funnel to pour the mixture into nail polish bottles or containers. Seal tightly.

Additional Tips:

● *Layering*: Apply multiple thin coats for an intensified glossy effect.

● *Oil Ratios*: Adjust jojoba and vitamin E oils for a shinier or more nourishing polish.

● *Avoid Thick Coats*: Apply thin layers to prevent smudging and ensure faster drying.

Caution:

● *Allergic Reactions*: Test a small amount on a patch of skin before using extensively to check for allergies to the ingredients.

Commercial Version:

Considerations:

● CREATING A COMMERCIAL version can cater to consumers seeking organic glossy nail polish.

● Enhancing the formula for durability and mass production suitability is advisable.

Additional Ingredients for Commercial Version:

● ORGANIC CASTOR OIL (1 teaspoon): Improves durability and shine.

● Mica Powder (1/4 teaspoon): Adds extra shimmer and sparkle for a commercial appeal.

Why these additional ingredients?

- *Organic Castor Oil*: Enhances durability and glossiness, suitable for commercial use.
- *Mica Powder*: Adds a subtle shimmer, making the polish visually appealing for consumers.

Shelf Life:

- HOMEMADE VERSION: Best used within 2-3 months for optimal quality.
- Commercial Version: Shelf life can extend to 6-12 months with added preservatives.

Packaging Tips:

- OPT FOR TRANSPARENT or clear bottles to showcase the glossy polish.
- Ensure clear labeling highlighting the organic, glossy, and natural aspects of the product.

Unique Selling Point (USP):

- PROMOTE THE POLISH as an organic, nourishing, and glossy option, appealing to consumers seeking a natural yet stunning finish for their nails.

Shimmering Metal: DIY Organic Metallic Nail Polish for Radiant Nails

Ingredients:

- Clear Organic Nail Polish (3 tablespoons): Serves as the base for the metallic polish.
- Organic Mica Powder (1 teaspoon): Adds shimmer and metallic effect naturally.
- Organic Jojoba Oil (1/2 teaspoon): Provides shine and nourishment for healthy nails.
- Organic Vitamin E Oil (1/4 teaspoon): Enhances the metallic sheen and nourishes nails.
- Organic Mineral Pigment Powder (1/2 teaspoon): Adds color depth and metallic hues.

Why these ingredients?

- *Clear Organic Nail Polish*: Acts as the base, ensuring adhesion and durability of the metallic finish.
- *Organic Mica Powder*: Adds shimmer and metallic effect naturally, without synthetic additives.
- *Organic Jojoba Oil*: Provides shine and nourishment for maintaining healthy nails.
- *Organic Vitamin E Oil*: Enhances the metallic sheen while nourishing nails.
- *Organic Mineral Pigment Powder*: Adds color depth and metallic hues without compromising organic integrity.

Tools:

- SMALL MIXING BOWL
- Mixing Spoon or Stick
- Small Funnel
- Nail Polish Bottles or Containers

Method:

Homemade Version:

- PREPARATION: ENSURE cleanliness of the mixing bowl and spoon.
  - Base Mix: Pour the clear organic nail polish into the mixing bowl.
  - Shimmering Additions: Add mica powder, mineral pigment powder, jojoba oil, and vitamin E oil. Mix thoroughly.
  - Consistency Check: Adjust pigment or clear polish for desired color intensity and consistency.
  - Bottling: Use a funnel to pour the mixture into nail polish bottles or containers. Seal tightly.

Additional Tips:

- *Layering*: Apply multiple coats for increased intensity and depth of the metallic effect.
  - *Experimentation*: Mix different pigment colors for unique metallic shades.
  - *Shake Before Use*: As natural ingredients might settle, shake the bottle before applying.

Caution:

- *Skin Sensitivity*: Before extensive use, test a small amount on a patch of skin to check for any allergic reactions to the ingredients.

Commercial Version:

Considerations:

- A COMMERCIAL VERSION of this metallic polish could attract consumers seeking organic, shimmering nail colors.
  - For commercial use, formulation adjustments for durability and mass production suitability are recommended.

Additional Ingredients for Commercial Version:

- ORGANIC CASTOR OIL (1 teaspoon): Enhances durability and glossiness for commercial use.
- Natural Preservative (as recommended for cosmetics): Extends shelf life for retail purposes.

Why these additional ingredients?

- *Organic Castor Oil*: Improves durability and glossiness, suitable for commercial distribution.
- *Natural Preservative*: Essential for retail sales, preventing bacterial growth and extending shelf life.

Shelf Life:

- HOMEMADE VERSION: Best used within 2-3 months for optimal quality.
- Commercial Version: With added preservatives, shelf life can extend to 6-12 months.

Packaging Tips:

- OPT FOR SLEEK AND attractive packaging that showcases the metallic polish.
- Clearly label the product as organic, metallic, and natural to appeal to eco-conscious consumers.

Unique Selling Point (USP):

- HIGHLIGHT THE POLISH as an organic, shimmering option for those wanting a natural yet glamorous metallic nail finish.

Sparkle Magic: DIY Organic Glitter Nail Polish for Dazzling Nails

Ingredients:

- Clear Organic Nail Polish (3 tablespoons): Acts as the base for the glittery polish.
- Organic Mica Powder (1 teaspoon): Adds shimmer and sparkle naturally.
- Organic Cosmetic-Grade Glitter (1/2 teaspoon): Provides glittery effects without harmful additives.
- Organic Jojoba Oil (1/2 teaspoon): Adds shine and nourishment for healthy nails.
- Organic Vitamin E Oil (1/4 teaspoon): Enhances the glittery effect and nourishes nails.

Why these ingredients?

- *Clear Organic Nail Polish*: Serves as the base, ensuring adhesion and durability of the glitter.
- *Organic Mica Powder*: Adds shimmer and sparkle organically without synthetic additives.
- *Organic Cosmetic-Grade Glitter*: Provides safe glittery effects without harmful substances.
- *Organic Jojoba Oil*: Adds shine and nourishment for maintaining healthy nails.
- *Organic Vitamin E Oil*: Enhances the glittery effect while nourishing nails.

Tools:

- SMALL MIXING BOWL
- Mixing Spoon or Stick
- Small Funnel
- Nail Polish Bottles or Containers

Method:

Homemade Version:

- PREPARATION: ENSURE cleanliness of the mixing bowl and spoon.
    - Base Mix: Pour the clear organic nail polish into the mixing bowl.
    - Sparkling Additions: Add mica powder, cosmetic-grade glitter, jojoba oil, and vitamin E oil. Mix thoroughly.
    - Consistency Check: Adjust glitter or clear polish for the desired sparkle and consistency.
    - Bottling: Use a funnel to pour the mixture into nail polish bottles or containers. Seal tightly.

Additional Tips:

- *Layering*: Apply multiple coats for increased intensity and depth of the glitter effect.
    - *Glitter Distribution*: To evenly distribute glitter, roll the bottle between your hands before use.
    - *Top Coat*: Apply a clear topcoat to seal and prolong the glittery effect.

Caution:

- *Skin Sensitivity*: Test a small amount on a patch of skin before extensive use to check for allergic reactions to the ingredients.

Commercial Version:

Considerations:

- A COMMERCIAL VERSION of this glitter polish might appeal to consumers seeking organic and glamorous nail colors.
    - Formulation adjustments for durability and mass production suitability are advisable.

Additional Ingredients for Commercial Version:

● ORGANIC CASTOR OIL (1 teaspoon): Enhances durability and sparkle for commercial use.

● Natural Preservative (as recommended for cosmetics): Extends shelf life for retail purposes.

Why these additional ingredients?

● *Organic Castor Oil*: Improves durability and sparkle, suitable for commercial distribution.

● *Natural Preservative*: Crucial for retail sales, preventing bacterial growth and extending shelf life.

Shelf Life:

● HOMEMADE VERSION: Best used within 2-3 months for optimal quality.

● Commercial Version: With added preservatives, shelf life can extend to 6-12 months.

Packaging Tips:

● OPT FOR APPEALING packaging that showcases the glittery polish.

● Clearly label the product as organic, glittery, and natural to attract environmentally conscious consumers.

Unique Selling Point (USP):

● HIGHLIGHT THE POLISH as an organic, dazzling option for those wanting a natural yet glamorous glitter nail finish.

Radiant Glow: DIY Organic Neon Nail Polish for Vibrant Nails

Ingredients:

- Clear Organic Nail Polish (3 tablespoons): Acts as the base for the neon polish.
- Organic Neon Pigment Powder (1 teaspoon): Provides vibrant and fluorescent colors naturally.
- Organic Jojoba Oil (1/2 teaspoon): Adds shine and nourishment for healthy nails.
- Organic Vitamin E Oil (1/4 teaspoon): Enhances the neon effect and nourishes nails.

Why these ingredients?

- *Clear Organic Nail Polish*: Serves as the base, ensuring adhesion and durability of the neon color.
- *Organic Neon Pigment Powder*: Offers vibrant and fluorescent colors without harmful additives.
- *Organic Jojoba Oil*: Adds shine and nourishment for maintaining healthy nails.
- *Organic Vitamin E Oil*: Enhances the neon effect while nourishing nails.

Tools:

- SMALL MIXING BOWL
- Mixing Spoon or Stick
- Small Funnel
- Nail Polish Bottles or Containers

Method:

Homemade Version:

PREPARATION: ENSURE cleanliness of the mixing bowl and spoon.

Base Mix: Pour the clear organic nail polish into the mixing bowl.

Neon Additions: Add neon pigment powder, jojoba oil, and vitamin E oil. Mix thoroughly.

Consistency Check: Adjust pigment or clear polish for the desired neon color and consistency.

Bottling: Use a funnel to pour the mixture into nail polish bottles or containers. Seal tightly.

Additional Tips:

- *Layering*: Apply multiple coats for intensified neon colors.
- *Color Mixing*: Experiment with different pigment ratios for unique neon shades.
- *Top Coat*: Apply a clear topcoat to seal and prolong the vibrant neon effect.

Caution:

- *Skin Sensitivity*: Test a small amount on a patch of skin before extensive use to check for allergic reactions to the ingredients.

Commercial Version:

Considerations:

- A COMMERCIAL VERSION of this neon polish might appeal to consumers seeking organic and vibrant nail colors.
- Adjustments for formulation durability and mass production suitability are advisable.

Additional Ingredients for Commercial Version:

- ORGANIC CASTOR OIL (1 teaspoon): Enhances durability and vibrancy for commercial use.
- Natural Preservative (as recommended for cosmetics): Extends shelf life for retail purposes.

Why these additional ingredients?

- *Organic Castor Oil*: Improves durability and vibrancy, suitable for commercial distribution.
- *Natural Preservative*: Essential for retail sales, preventing bacterial growth and extending shelf life.

Shelf Life:

- HOMEMADE VERSION: Best used within 2-3 months for optimal quality.
- Commercial Version: With added preservatives, shelf life can extend to 6-12 months.

Packaging Tips:

- OPT FOR EYE-CATCHING packaging that showcases the vibrant neon polish.
- Clearly label the product as organic, neon, and natural to attract environmentally conscious consumers.

Unique Selling Point (USP):

- HIGHLIGHT THE POLISH as an organic, vibrant option for those seeking a natural yet bold neon nail finish.

Color Shift Charm: DIY Organic Thermal Nail Polish for Magical Effects

Ingredients:

- Clear Organic Nail Polish (3 tablespoons): Acts as the base for the thermal polish.
- Organic Thermal Pigment Powder (1 teaspoon): Provides color change based on temperature.
- Organic Jojoba Oil (1/2 teaspoon): Adds shine and nourishment for healthy nails.
- Organic Vitamin E Oil (1/4 teaspoon): Enhances the thermal effect and nourishes nails.

Why these ingredients?

- *Clear Organic Nail Polish*: Serves as the base, ensuring adhesion and durability of the thermal effect.
- *Organic Thermal Pigment Powder*: Responsible for the color change based on temperature without harmful additives.
- *Organic Jojoba Oil*: Adds shine and nourishment for maintaining healthy nails.
- *Organic Vitamin E Oil*: Enhances the thermal effect while nourishing nails.

Tools:

- SMALL MIXING BOWL
- Mixing Spoon or Stick
- Small Funnel
- Nail Polish Bottles or Containers

Method:

Homemade Version:

- PREPARATION: ENSURE cleanliness of the mixing bowl and spoon.

- Base Mix: Pour the clear organic nail polish into the mixing bowl.
- Thermal Additions: Add thermal pigment powder, jojoba oil, and vitamin E oil. Mix thoroughly.
- Consistency Check: Adjust pigment or clear polish for the desired thermal effect and consistency.
- Bottling: Use a funnel to pour the mixture into nail polish bottles or containers. Seal tightly.

Additional Tips:

- *Temperature Variance*: Test the color shift by placing nails under warm and cold water.
- *Layering*: Apply multiple coats for intensified color change.
- *Top Coat*: Apply a clear topcoat to seal and prolong the thermal effect.

Caution:

- *Skin Sensitivity*: Test a small amount on a patch of skin before extensive use to check for allergic reactions to the ingredients.

Commercial Version:

Considerations:

- A COMMERCIAL VERSION of this thermal polish might interest consumers seeking organic and innovative nail colors.
- Formulation adjustments for durability and mass production suitability are advisable.

Additional Ingredients for Commercial Version:

- ORGANIC CASTOR OIL (1 teaspoon): Enhances durability and thermal effects for commercial use.
- Natural Preservative (as recommended for cosmetics): Extends shelf life for retail purposes.

Why these additional ingredients?

- *Organic Castor Oil*: Improves durability and thermal effects, suitable for commercial distribution.
- *Natural Preservative*: Essential for retail sales, preventing bacterial growth and extending shelf life.

Shelf Life:

- HOMEMADE VERSION: Best used within 2-3 months for optimal quality.
- Commercial Version: With added preservatives, shelf life can extend to 6-12 months.

Packaging Tips:

- CHOOSE PACKAGING that showcases the color shift of the thermal polish.
- Clearly label the product as organic, thermal, and natural to appeal to eco-conscious consumers.

Unique Selling Point (USP):

- EMPHASIZE THE POLISH as an organic, innovative option for those desiring a natural yet mesmerizing thermal effect on their nails.

Peel Away Glam: DIY Organic Peelable Nail Polish for Easy Removal

Ingredients:

- Clear Organic Nail Polish (3 tablespoons): Serves as the base for the peelable polish.
- Organic Cornstarch (2 teaspoons): Adds peelability without harmful chemicals.
- Organic Glycerin (1 teaspoon): Enhances flexibility for easy peeling.
- Organic Vitamin E Oil (1/4 teaspoon): Nourishes nails while maintaining peelability.

Why these ingredients?

- *Clear Organic Nail Polish*: Base for the peelable polish, ensuring adhesion.
- *Organic Cornstarch*: Provides peelability without resorting to harmful substances.
- *Organic Glycerin*: Adds flexibility, aiding in the easy removal of the polish.
- *Organic Vitamin E Oil*: Nourishes nails while maintaining peelability and nail health.

Tools:

- SMALL MIXING BOWL
  - Mixing Spoon or Stick
  - Small Funnel
  - Nail Polish Bottles or Containers

Method:

Homemade Version:

- PREPARATION: ENSURE cleanliness of the mixing bowl and spoon.
  - Base Mix: Pour the clear organic nail polish into the mixing bowl.

• Peelable Additions: Add cornstarch, glycerin, and vitamin E oil. Mix thoroughly.

• Consistency Check: Adjust ingredients for desired consistency for easy application.

• Bottling: Use a funnel to pour the mixture into nail polish bottles or containers. Seal tightly.

Additional Tips:

• *Thin Layers*: Apply thin coats for better peelability.

• *Drying Time*: Allow each layer to dry thoroughly before applying the next.

• *Peeling Technique*: Start peeling from the cuticle area for easier removal.

Caution:

• *Skin Sensitivity*: Test a small amount on a patch of skin before extensive use to check for allergic reactions to the ingredients.

Commercial Version:

Considerations:

• CREATING A COMMERCIAL version of this peelable polish can attract consumers seeking an easy and organic nail polish removal option.

• Formulation adjustments for durability and mass production suitability are recommended.

Additional Ingredients for Commercial Version:

• ORGANIC TAPIOCA Starch (1 teaspoon): Enhances peelability for commercial distribution.

• Natural Preservative (as recommended for cosmetics): Extends shelf life for retail purposes.

Why these additional ingredients?

- *Organic Tapioca Starch*: Improves peelability, suitable for commercial use.
- *Natural Preservative*: Crucial for retail sales, preventing bacterial growth and extending shelf life.

Shelf Life:

- HOMEMADE VERSION: Best used within 2-3 months for optimal quality.
- Commercial Version: With added preservatives, shelf life can extend to 6-12 months.

Packaging Tips:

- USE CLEAR LABELING to highlight the peelable and organic aspects of the polish.
- Consider packaging that indicates the ease of removal as a unique feature.

Unique Selling Point (USP):

- MARKET THE POLISH as an organic, hassle-free option for easy removal, appealing to those wanting a convenient and gentle nail polish experience.

Crackling Craze: DIY Organic Crackle Nail Polish for Unique Designs

Ingredients:

- Clear Organic Nail Polish (3 tablespoons): Serves as the base for the crackle effect.
- Organic Cornstarch (1 teaspoon): Aids in crackling when applied over the base polish.
- Organic Glycerin (1/2 teaspoon): Enhances flexibility for better crackle patterns.
- Organic Vitamin E Oil (1/4 teaspoon): Nourishes nails while allowing crackling.

Why these ingredients?

- *Clear Organic Nail Polish*: Base for the crackle effect, ensuring adhesion.
- *Organic Cornstarch*: Aids in crackling when applied over the base polish.
- *Organic Glycerin*: Adds flexibility, aiding in crackle pattern formation.
- *Organic Vitamin E Oil*: Nourishes nails while enabling crackling.

Tools:

- SMALL MIXING BOWL
  - Mixing Spoon or Stick
  - Small Funnel
  - Nail Polish Bottles or Containers

Method:

Homemade Version:

PREPARATION: ENSURE cleanliness of the mixing bowl and spoon.

Base Mix: Pour the clear organic nail polish into the mixing bowl.

Crackle Additions: Add cornstarch, glycerin, and vitamin E oil. Mix thoroughly.

Consistency Check: Ensure the mixture is smooth and consistent.

Bottling: Use a funnel to pour the mixture into nail polish bottles or containers. Seal tightly.

Additional Tips:

● *Quick Application*: Apply the crackle polish thinly and swiftly for better crackling.

● *Contrast Colors*: Use contrasting base and crackle colors for striking designs.

● *Top Coat*: Apply a clear topcoat to seal and protect the crackle design.

Caution:

● *Skin Sensitivity*: Test a small amount on a patch of skin before extensive use to check for allergic reactions to the ingredients.

Commercial Version:

Considerations:

● A COMMERCIAL VERSION of this crackle polish might appeal to consumers seeking organic and trendy nail art options.

● Adjustments for formulation durability and mass production suitability are recommended.

Additional Ingredients for Commercial Version:

● ORGANIC KAOLIN CLAY (1/2 teaspoon): Enhances crackle patterns for commercial distribution.

● Natural Preservative (as recommended for cosmetics): Extends shelf life for retail purposes.

Why these additional ingredients?

● *Organic Kaolin Clay*: Improves crackle patterns, suitable for commercial use.

- *Natural Preservative*: Essential for retail sales, preventing bacterial growth and extending shelf life.

Shelf Life:

- HOMEMADE VERSION: Best used within 2-3 months for optimal quality.
- Commercial Version: With added preservatives, shelf life can extend to 6-12 months.

Packaging Tips:

- USE CLEAR LABELING to highlight the crackle effect and organic nature of the polish.
- Consider packaging that showcases the crackle pattern as a unique feature.

Unique Selling Point (USP):

- MARKET THE POLISH as an organic, artful option for those seeking trendy and innovative nail designs through crackling techniques.

Morph Magic: DIY Organic Chameleon Nail Polish for Shifting Hues

Ingredients:

- Clear Organic Nail Polish (3 tablespoons): Serves as the base for the chameleon effect.
- Organic Chameleon Pigment Powder (1 teaspoon): Provides color-shifting properties.
- Organic Jojoba Oil (1/2 teaspoon): Adds shine and nourishment for healthy nails.
- Organic Vitamin E Oil (1/4 teaspoon): Enhances the chameleon effect and nourishes nails.

Why these ingredients?

- *Clear Organic Nail Polish*: Base for the chameleon effect, ensuring adhesion.
- *Organic Chameleon Pigment Powder*: Offers color-shifting properties without harmful additives.
- *Organic Jojoba Oil*: Adds shine and nourishment for maintaining healthy nails.
- *Organic Vitamin E Oil*: Enhances the chameleon effect while nourishing nails.

Tools:

- SMALL MIXING BOWL
  - Mixing Spoon or Stick
  - Small Funnel
  - Nail Polish Bottles or Containers

Method:

Homemade Version:

PREPARATION: ENSURE cleanliness of the mixing bowl and spoon.

Base Mix: Pour the clear organic nail polish into the mixing bowl.

Chameleon Additions: Add chameleon pigment powder, jojoba oil, and vitamin E oil. Mix thoroughly.

Consistency Check: Ensure the mixture is smooth and consistent.

Bottling: Use a funnel to pour the mixture into nail polish bottles or containers. Seal tightly.

Additional Tips:

- *Thin Layers*: Apply thin coats for better color shifting.
- *Lighting Effects*: Observe the color shift under different lighting conditions.
- *Top Coat*: Apply a clear topcoat to seal and prolong the chameleon effect.

Caution:

- *Skin Sensitivity*: Test a small amount on a patch of skin before extensive use to check for allergic reactions to the ingredients.

Commercial Version:

Considerations:

- A COMMERCIAL VERSION of this chameleon polish might attract consumers seeking organic and innovative nail colors.
- Adjustments for formulation durability and mass production suitability are recommended.

Additional Ingredients for Commercial Version:

- ORGANIC SILICA (1/2 teaspoon): Enhances color-shifting effects for commercial distribution.
- Natural Preservative (as recommended for cosmetics): Extends shelf life for retail purposes.

Why these additional ingredients?

- *Organic Silica*: Improves color-shifting effects, suitable for commercial use.
- *Natural Preservative*: Crucial for retail sales, preventing bacterial growth and extending shelf life.

Shelf Life:

- HOMEMADE VERSION: Best used within 2-3 months for optimal quality.
- Commercial Version: With added preservatives, shelf life can extend to 6-12 months.

Packaging Tips:

- USE CLEAR LABELING to highlight the chameleon effect and organic nature of the polish.
- Consider packaging that showcases the color-shifting ability as a unique feature.

Unique Selling Point (USP):

- MARKET THE POLISH as an organic, mesmerizing option for those seeking an innovative and constantly shifting hue on their nails through the chameleon effect.

Fragrant Whiffs: DIY Organic Scented Nail Polish for Aromatherapy Glam

Ingredients:

- Clear Organic Nail Polish (3 tablespoons): Base for the scented polish.
- Organic Essential Oil (10-15 drops): Adds fragrance to the nail polish.
- Organic Jojoba Oil (1/2 teaspoon): Enhances nail health and fragrance diffusion.
- Organic Vitamin E Oil (1/4 teaspoon): Nourishes nails while maintaining scent.

Why these ingredients?

- *Clear Organic Nail Polish*: Base for the scented polish, ensuring adhesion.
- *Organic Essential Oil*: Adds natural fragrance without harmful chemicals.
- *Organic Jojoba Oil*: Enhances fragrance diffusion and nail health.
- *Organic Vitamin E Oil*: Nourishes nails while maintaining scent and nail health.

Tools:

- SMALL MIXING BOWL
- Mixing Spoon or Stick
- Small Funnel
- Nail Polish Bottles or Containers

Method:

Homemade Version:

PREPARATION: ENSURE cleanliness of the mixing bowl and spoon.

Base Mix: Pour the clear organic nail polish into the mixing bowl.

Fragrance Addition: Add essential oil, jojoba oil, and vitamin E oil. Mix thoroughly.

Consistency Check: Ensure the mixture is smooth and consistent.

Bottling: Use a funnel to pour the mixture into nail polish bottles or containers. Seal tightly.

Additional Tips:

● *Scent Strength*: Adjust the number of drops of essential oil for desired fragrance intensity.

● *Layering*: Apply multiple coats for increased fragrance effect.

● *Top Coat*: Apply a clear topcoat to seal and protect the scent.

Caution:

● *Skin Sensitivity*: Test a small amount on a patch of skin before extensive use to check for allergic reactions to the ingredients.

Commercial Version:

Considerations:

● A COMMERCIAL VERSION of scented polish can appeal to consumers seeking both beauty and aromatherapy benefits.

● Formulation adjustments for durability and mass production suitability are advisable.

Additional Ingredients for Commercial Version:

● ORGANIC SOY WAX (1/2 teaspoon): Enhances scent retention for commercial distribution.

● Natural Preservative (as recommended for cosmetics): Extends shelf life for retail purposes.

Why these additional ingredients?

● *Organic Soy Wax*: Improves scent retention, suitable for commercial use.

● *Natural Preservative*: Essential for retail sales, preventing bacterial growth and extending shelf life.

Shelf Life:

● HOMEMADE VERSION: Best used within 2-3 months for optimal quality.

● Commercial Version: With added preservatives, shelf life can extend to 6-12 months.

Packaging Tips:

● CHOOSE PACKAGING that preserves the scent and highlights the organic, aromatherapy aspect of the polish.

● Clearly label the product as scented, organic, and suitable for aromatherapy.

Unique Selling Point (USP):

● MARKET THE POLISH as an organic, scented option for those desiring both a glamorous nail look and the therapeutic benefits of aromatherapy.

Shimmering Illusions: DIY Organic Holographic Nail Polish for Dazzling Nails

Ingredients:

- Clear Organic Nail Polish (3 tablespoons): Base for the holographic effect.
- Organic Holographic Pigment Powder (1 teaspoon): Provides holographic shimmer.
- Organic Jojoba Oil (1/2 teaspoon): Enhances nail health and holographic dispersion.
- Organic Vitamin E Oil (1/4 teaspoon): Nourishes nails while maintaining holographic shine.

Why these ingredients?

- *Clear Organic Nail Polish*: Base for the holographic effect, ensuring adhesion.
- *Organic Holographic Pigment Powder*: Adds holographic shimmer without harmful additives.
- *Organic Jojoba Oil*: Enhances holographic dispersion while nourishing nails.
- *Organic Vitamin E Oil*: Nourishes nails while maintaining holographic shine and nail health.

Tools:

- SMALL MIXING BOWL
- Mixing Spoon or Stick
- Small Funnel
- Nail Polish Bottles or Containers

Method:

Homemade Version:

PREPARATION: ENSURE cleanliness of the mixing bowl and spoon.

Base Mix: Pour the clear organic nail polish into the mixing bowl.

Holographic Addition: Add holographic pigment powder, jojoba oil, and vitamin E oil. Mix thoroughly.

Consistency Check: Ensure the mixture is smooth and consistent.

Bottling: Use a funnel to pour the mixture into nail polish bottles or containers. Seal tightly.

Additional Tips:

- *Lighting Effects*: Observe the holographic effect under different lighting conditions.
- *Layering*: Apply multiple coats for intensified holographic shine.
- *Top Coat*: Apply a clear topcoat to seal and protect the holographic effect.

Caution:

- *Skin Sensitivity*: Test a small amount on a patch of skin before extensive use to check for allergic reactions to the ingredients.

Commercial Version:

Considerations:

- A COMMERCIAL VERSION of holographic polish can attract consumers seeking both organic and trendy nail colors.
- Formulation adjustments for durability and mass production suitability are advisable.

Additional Ingredients for Commercial Version:

- ORGANIC MICA POWDER (1/2 teaspoon): Enhances holographic brilliance for commercial distribution.
- Natural Preservative (as recommended for cosmetics): Extends shelf life for retail purposes.

Why these additional ingredients?

- *Organic Mica Powder*: Improves holographic brilliance, suitable for commercial use.
- *Natural Preservative*: Crucial for retail sales, preventing bacterial growth and extending shelf life.

Shelf Life:

- HOMEMADE VERSION: Best used within 2-3 months for optimal quality.
- Commercial Version: With added preservatives, shelf life can extend to 6-12 months.

Packaging Tips:

- CHOOSE PACKAGING that emphasizes the holographic effect and organic nature of the polish.
- Clearly label the product as holographic, organic, and suitable for glamorous nail looks.

Unique Selling Point (USP):

- MARKET THE POLISH as an organic, radiant option for those seeking an enchanting holographic effect on their nails, without compromising on organic ingredients.

Textured Elegance: DIY Organic Textured Nail Polish for Unique Nails

Ingredients:

- Clear Organic Nail Polish (3 tablespoons): Base for the textured effect.
  - Organic Sugar (1 teaspoon): Adds granular texture to the polish.
- Organic Mica Powder (1/2 teaspoon): Enhances shimmer in the textured finish.
  - Organic Jojoba Oil (1/2 teaspoon): Nourishes nails and aids in texture adhesion.

Why these ingredients?

- *Clear Organic Nail Polish*: Base for the textured effect, ensuring adhesion.
- *Organic Sugar*: Provides granular texture without harmful additives.
- *Organic Mica Powder*: Enhances shimmer within the textured finish.
- *Organic Jojoba Oil*: Nourishes nails while aiding in texture adhesion.

Tools:

- SMALL MIXING BOWL
  - Mixing Spoon or Stick
  - Small Funnel
  - Nail Polish Bottles or Containers

Method:

Homemade Version:

PREPARATION: ENSURE cleanliness of the mixing bowl and spoon.

Base Mix: Pour the clear organic nail polish into the mixing bowl.

Texture Addition: Add sugar, mica powder, and jojoba oil. Mix thoroughly until the sugar dissolves slightly.

Consistency Check: Ensure the mixture has a textured yet spreadable consistency.

Bottling: Use a funnel to pour the mixture into nail polish bottles or containers. Seal tightly.

Additional Tips:

- *Texture Intensity*: Adjust the amount of sugar for varied levels of texture.
  - *Layering*: Experiment with layering coats for different textured effects.
  - *Top Coat*: Apply a clear topcoat to seal and protect the textured finish.

Caution:

- *Skin Sensitivity*: Test a small amount on a patch of skin before extensive use to check for allergic reactions to the ingredients.

Commercial Version:

Considerations:

- A COMMERCIAL VERSION of textured polish might intrigue consumers looking for organic and creative nail finishes.
  - Adjustments for formulation durability and mass production suitability are recommended.

Additional Ingredients for Commercial Version:

- ORGANIC SILICA POWDER (1/2 teaspoon): Enhances texture for commercial distribution.
  - Natural Preservative (as recommended for cosmetics): Extends shelf life for retail purposes.

  Why these additional ingredients?
  - *Organic Silica Powder*: Improves texture for commercial use.
  - *Natural Preservative*: Essential for retail sales, preventing bacterial growth and extending shelf life.

Shelf Life:

- HOMEMADE VERSION: Best used within 2-3 months for optimal quality.
    - Commercial Version: With added preservatives, shelf life can extend to 6-12 months.

Packaging Tips:

- OPT FOR PACKAGING that showcases the unique textured effect of the polish.
    - Clearly label the product as textured, organic, and suitable for creative nail designs.

Unique Selling Point (USP):

- MARKET THE POLISH as an organic, textured option for those seeking a unique and innovative look for their nails, while prioritizing organic ingredients.

Easy Peel: DIY Organic Peel-Off Base Coat for Gentle Nail Care

Ingredients:

- Organic Gelatin Powder (1 tablespoon): Creates the peel-off texture.
- Organic Aloe Vera Gel (1 tablespoon): Nourishes and strengthens nails.
- Organic Vegetable Glycerin (1/2 teaspoon): Adds flexibility to the base coat.
- Organic Lavender Essential Oil (3-4 drops): Provides a pleasant fragrance and aids in nail care.

Why these ingredients?

- *Organic Gelatin Powder*: Creates the peel-off texture without harmful chemicals.
- *Organic Aloe Vera Gel*: Nourishes and strengthens nails, promoting healthier nails.
- *Organic Vegetable Glycerin*: Adds flexibility to the base coat for easy peeling.
- *Organic Lavender Essential Oil*: Offers a pleasant fragrance while providing additional nail care benefits.

Tools:

- SMALL MIXING BOWL
  - Mixing Spoon or Stick
  - Small Funnel
  - Nail Polish Bottles or Containers

Method:

Homemade Version:

PREPARATION: ENSURE cleanliness of the mixing bowl and spoon.

Base Mix: Combine organic gelatin powder and aloe vera gel in the mixing bowl. Stir well until smooth.

Additional Ingredients: Add vegetable glycerin and lavender essential oil. Mix thoroughly.

Consistency Check: Ensure the mixture has a smooth, slightly runny consistency.

Bottling: Use a funnel to pour the mixture into nail polish bottles or containers. Seal tightly.

Additional Tips:

- *Thin Layers*: Apply thin coats for better peelability.
  - *Dry Time*: Allow each layer to dry completely before applying the next.
  - *Removal*: Gently lift the edges of the base coat to peel it off easily.

Caution:

- *Skin Sensitivity*: Perform a patch test on a small area of skin before use to check for allergies to the ingredients.

Commercial Version:

Considerations:

- CREATING A COMMERCIAL version of peel-off base coat might appeal to consumers seeking organic and gentle nail care options.
  - Modifications for formulation durability and mass production suitability are advisable.

Additional Ingredients for Commercial Version:

- NATURAL PRESERVATIVE (as recommended for cosmetics): Enhances shelf life for retail purposes.
  - Why this additional ingredient?
  - *Natural Preservative*: Essential for retail sales, preventing bacterial growth and extending shelf life.

Shelf Life:

- HOMEMADE VERSION: Best used within 1-2 months for optimal quality.
  - Commercial Version: With added preservatives, shelf life can extend to 6-12 months.

Packaging Tips:

- CHOOSE PACKAGING that highlights the peel-off nature and organic properties of the base coat.
  - Clearly label the product as a peel-off base coat, emphasizing its organic formulation.

Unique Selling Point (USP):

- MARKET THE BASE coat as an organic, gentle alternative for those seeking a hassle-free, nail-friendly way to remove nail polish.

Gentle Cleanse: Organic DIY Acetone-Free Nail Polish Remover

Ingredients:

- Organic Apple Cider Vinegar (3 tablespoons): Helps soften and dissolve nail polish.
- Organic Lemon Essential Oil (5-6 drops): Adds natural cleansing properties and a fresh scent.
- Organic Glycerin (1 tablespoon): Moisturizes nails and cuticles during the removal process.
- Distilled Water (3 tablespoons): Dilutes the solution for gentler action.

Why these ingredients?

- *Organic Apple Cider Vinegar*: Softens and dissolves nail polish gently.
- *Organic Lemon Essential Oil*: Provides cleansing properties without harsh chemicals.
- *Organic Glycerin*: Moisturizes nails and cuticles to counteract dryness.
- *Distilled Water*: Dilutes the solution for a milder, yet effective, nail polish removal.

Tools:

- SMALL MIXING BOWL
- Mixing Spoon or Stick
- Small Funnel
- Airtight Glass Container or Bottle

Method:

Homemade Version:

PREPARATION: ENSURE cleanliness of the mixing bowl and utensils.

Mixing: Combine organic apple cider vinegar, lemon essential oil, glycerin, and distilled water in the mixing bowl. Stir well until thoroughly mixed.

Transfer: Use a funnel to pour the mixture into an airtight glass container or bottle for storage.

Additional Tips:

- *Soak Time*: Allow the remover to sit on nails for a few seconds before wiping off to help dissolve polish effectively.
- *Gentle Patting*: Rather than rubbing vigorously, gently pat the nails to remove dissolved polish.

Caution:

- *Skin Sensitivity*: Test a small amount on a patch of skin before extensive use to check for any allergic reactions to the ingredients.

Commercial Version:

Considerations:

- CREATING A COMMERCIAL version of acetone-free nail polish remover can appeal to consumers seeking organic and gentle nail care options.
- Modifications for formulation durability and mass production suitability are advisable.

Additional Ingredients for Commercial Version:

- NATURAL PRESERVATIVE (as recommended for cosmetics): Enhances shelf life for retail purposes.
  Why this additional ingredient?
- *Natural Preservative*: Crucial for retail sales, preventing bacterial growth and extending shelf life.

Shelf Life:

- HOMEMADE VERSION: Best used within 1-2 months for optimal quality.

- Commercial Version: With added preservatives, shelf life can extend to 6-12 months.

Packaging Tips:

- CHOOSE A GLASS OR recyclable plastic packaging to emphasize eco-friendliness.
- Clearly label the product as acetone-free, organic, and suitable for gentle nail polish removal.

Unique Selling Point (USP):

- MARKET THE REMOVER as an organic, gentle alternative for nail polish removal, free from harsh chemicals typically found in traditional removers.

Citrus Refresh: Organic Lemon and Vinegar Nail Polish Remover

Ingredients:

- Organic Lemon Juice (3 tablespoons): Contains natural acids to dissolve polish.
- Organic White Vinegar (3 tablespoons): Acts as a solvent to remove nail polish.
- Organic Olive Oil (1 tablespoon): Nourishes and moisturizes nails and cuticles.
- Distilled Water (3 tablespoons): Dilutes the solution for a gentler action.

Why these ingredients?

- *Organic Lemon Juice*: Natural acids effectively dissolve nail polish without harsh chemicals.
- *Organic White Vinegar*: Acts as a solvent to break down and remove nail polish gently.
- *Organic Olive Oil*: Nourishes nails and cuticles, counteracting dryness during the removal process.
- *Distilled Water*: Dilutes the solution for a milder yet effective nail polish removal.

Tools:

- SMALL MIXING BOWL
  - Mixing Spoon or Stick
  - Small Funnel
  - Airtight Glass Container or Bottle

Method:

Homemade Version:

- PREPARATION: ENSURE cleanliness of the mixing bowl and utensils.

- Mixing: Combine organic lemon juice, white vinegar, olive oil, and distilled water in the mixing bowl. Stir well until thoroughly mixed.
- Transfer: Use a funnel to pour the mixture into an airtight glass container or bottle for storage.

Additional Tips:

- *Soak Time*: Allow the remover to sit on nails for a few seconds before wiping off to dissolve polish effectively.
- *Gentle Patting*: Instead of rubbing vigorously, gently pat the nails to remove dissolved polish.

Caution:

- *Skin Sensitivity*: Always perform a patch test on a small area of skin before extensive use to check for any allergic reactions to the ingredients.

Commercial Version:

Considerations:

- CREATING A COMMERCIAL version of lemon and vinegar nail polish remover can attract consumers seeking organic and natural nail care options.
- Modifications for formulation durability and mass production suitability are advisable.

Additional Ingredients for Commercial Version:

- NATURAL PRESERVATIVE (as recommended for cosmetics): Enhances shelf life for retail purposes.
  Why this additional ingredient?
- *Natural Preservative*: Crucial for retail sales, preventing bacterial growth and extending shelf life.

Shelf Life:

- HOMEMADE VERSION: Best used within 1-2 months for optimal quality.
  - Commercial Version: With added preservatives, shelf life can extend to 6-12 months.

Packaging Tips:

- CHOOSE ECO-FRIENDLY packaging materials, such as glass or recyclable plastic, to emphasize sustainability.
  - Clearly label the product as an organic, lemon, and vinegar-based nail polish remover.

Unique Selling Point (USP):

- MARKET THE REMOVER as an organic, citrus-infused solution for gentle and effective nail polish removal, offering a refreshing twist on traditional removers.

Pure Cleanse: Organic Rubbing Alcohol Nail Polish Remover

Ingredients:

- Organic Rubbing Alcohol (3 tablespoons): Acts as a solvent to dissolve and remove nail polish.
- Organic Glycerin (1 tablespoon): Moisturizes and protects nails and cuticles.
- Organic Lavender Essential Oil (5-6 drops): Adds a pleasant scent and offers nail care benefits.
- Distilled Water (2 tablespoons): Dilutes the solution for a gentler action.

Why these ingredients?

- *Organic Rubbing Alcohol*: Acts as a solvent to effectively dissolve nail polish without harsh chemicals.
- *Organic Glycerin*: Moisturizes and protects nails, counteracting dryness during the removal process.
- *Organic Lavender Essential Oil*: Provides a pleasant fragrance and additional nail care benefits.
- *Distilled Water*: Dilutes the solution for a milder yet effective nail polish removal.

Tools:

- SMALL MIXING BOWL
- Mixing Spoon or Stick
- Small Funnel
- Airtight Glass Container or Bottle

Method:

Homemade Version:

- PREPARATION: ENSURE cleanliness of the mixing bowl and utensils.

● Mixing: Combine organic rubbing alcohol, glycerin, lavender essential oil, and distilled water in the mixing bowl. Stir well until thoroughly mixed.

● Transfer: Use a funnel to pour the mixture into an airtight glass container or bottle for storage.

Additional Tips:

● *Cotton Pad Usage*: Apply the solution to a cotton pad and gently press it onto the nail for a few seconds before wiping off.

● *Gentle Wiping*: Instead of rubbing vigorously, gently wipe off the dissolved polish.

Caution:

● *Flammability*: Store the solution away from heat sources and flames due to the alcohol content.

● *Skin Sensitivity*: Perform a patch test on a small area of skin before extensive use to check for any allergic reactions to the ingredients.

Commercial Version:

Considerations:

● CREATING A COMMERCIAL version of rubbing alcohol nail polish remover can appeal to consumers seeking organic and effective nail care solutions.

● Modifications for formulation durability and mass production suitability are advisable.

Additional Ingredients for Commercial Version:

● NATURAL PRESERVATIVE (as recommended for cosmetics): Enhances shelf life for retail purposes.

Why this additional ingredient?

● *Natural Preservative*: Crucial for retail sales, preventing bacterial growth and extending shelf life.

Shelf Life:

• HOMEMADE VERSION: Best used within 1-2 months for optimal quality.

• Commercial Version: With added preservatives, shelf life can extend to 6-12 months.

Packaging Tips:

• OPT FOR STURDY, airtight glass or recyclable plastic packaging for safety and sustainability.

• Clearly label the product as an organic, alcohol-based nail polish remover.

Unique Selling Point (USP):

• MARKET THE REMOVER as an organic, alcohol-based solution for effective nail polish removal without the use of harsh chemicals.

Easy Swipe: Organic DIY Nail Polish Remover Pads

Ingredients:

- Organic Cotton Pads (10 pads): Provides the base for the remover pads.
- Organic Rubbing Alcohol (2 tablespoons): Acts as a solvent to dissolve nail polish.
- Organic Glycerin (1 tablespoon): Moisturizes and protects nails and cuticles.
- Organic Lavender Essential Oil (8-10 drops): Adds a pleasant scent and offers nail care benefits.

Why these ingredients?

- *Organic Cotton Pads*: Serve as the base for the remover pads, gentle on the skin.
- *Organic Rubbing Alcohol*: Acts as a solvent to effectively remove nail polish.
- *Organic Glycerin*: Provides moisture to prevent dryness during the removal process.
- *Organic Lavender Essential Oil*: Adds a pleasing aroma and additional nail care properties.

Tools:

- SMALL AIRTIGHT CONTAINER or Jar
- Mixing Bowl or Plate
- Tweezers or Small Tongs (optional)

Method:

Homemade Version:

PREPARATION: LAY OUT the organic cotton pads on a clean surface.

Mixing: In a mixing bowl or plate, combine organic rubbing alcohol, glycerin, and lavender essential oil. Stir well to ensure even distribution.

Soaking: Dip each cotton pad into the mixture, allowing it to absorb the solution. Ensure each pad is thoroughly soaked but not dripping.

Stacking: Carefully stack the soaked pads in a small airtight container or jar. Use tweezers or small tongs if needed to avoid getting the solution on your hands.

Sealing: Seal the container or jar tightly to prevent the pads from drying out.

Additional Tips:

- *Pad Thickness*: For a thicker pad, use multiple cotton pads stacked together.
  - *Storage*: Store the container or jar in a cool, dry place away from direct sunlight to preserve the effectiveness of the pads.

Caution:

- *Flammability*: Store the pads away from heat sources and flames due to the alcohol content.
  - *Skin Sensitivity*: Perform a patch test on a small area of skin before extensive use to check for any allergic reactions to the ingredients.

Commercial Version:

Considerations:

- CREATING A COMMERCIAL version of DIY nail polish remover pads can cater to consumers seeking convenient and organic nail care options.
  - Modifications for formulation durability and mass production suitability are advisable.

Additional Ingredients for Commercial Version:

- NATURAL PRESERVATIVE (as recommended for cosmetics): Enhances shelf life for retail purposes.

Why this additional ingredient?

● *Natural Preservative*: Crucial for retail sales, preventing bacterial growth and extending shelf life.

Shelf Life:

● HOMEMADE VERSION: Best used within 1-2 months for optimal quality.

● Commercial Version: With added preservatives, shelf life can extend to 6-12 months.

Packaging Tips:

● USE ENVIRONMENTALLY-friendly packaging materials, such as recyclable jars or containers.

● Clearly label the product as organic, alcohol-based nail polish remover pads.

Unique Selling Point (USP):

● MARKET THE PADS as a convenient, on-the-go solution for quick and organic nail polish removal, emphasizing their natural and gentle composition.

Soothing Aloe Vera Primer for Natural Glow

Ingredients:

- Aloe Vera Gel (3 tablespoons): A natural moisturizer, it hydrates the skin without clogging pores, creating a smooth base for makeup.
- Coconut Oil (1 teaspoon): Provides a light barrier to lock in moisture and offers antimicrobial properties, keeping the skin healthy.
- Glycerin (1 teaspoon, optional): Enhances the primer's moisturizing effect, leaving the skin supple and soft.
- Lavender Essential Oil (1-2 drops): Offers a delicate fragrance and possesses calming properties for the skin.

Description of Ingredients:

- Aloe Vera Gel: Known for its healing properties, aloe vera gel soothes and hydrates the skin, perfect for a primer base.
- Coconut Oil: Provides a light, non-greasy layer that moisturizes and protects the skin while preventing makeup from settling into fine lines.
- Glycerin: Acts as a humectant, drawing moisture to the skin's surface, promoting hydration.
- Lavender Essential Oil: Adds a pleasant scent while possessing calming effects on the skin.

Tools Required:

- Mixing Bowl
- Spoon or Whisk
- Small Airtight Container for Storage

Method:

Homemade Version:

COMBINE INGREDIENTS: In a mixing bowl, blend 3 tablespoons of aloe vera gel, 1 teaspoon of coconut oil, and optionally, 1 teaspoon of glycerin.

Add Essential Oil: Drop in 1-2 drops of lavender essential oil and mix thoroughly.

Transfer to Container: Pour the mixture into a small airtight container suitable for storage.

Additional Tips:

• Conduct a patch test on a small area of skin to ensure no allergic reactions occur.

• Adjust the amount of essential oil to suit personal preferences for fragrance intensity.

• Store the primer in a cool, dry place away from direct sunlight for longevity.

Caution:

• Discontinue use if any irritation or discomfort occurs.

• Avoid getting the mixture into the eyes.

Commercial Version:

CREATING A COMMERCIAL version of this primer requires adherence to specific regulations. For commercial production:

• It's advisable to use organic ingredients certified for cosmetic use.

• Additional stabilizers or preservatives might be necessary for a longer shelf life, such as vitamin E oil or a natural preservative like grapefruit seed extract.

• Commercial packaging should ensure hygiene and preservation of the product's integrity.

- Shelf life can vary but may typically range from 6 to 12 months, depending on preservatives used.
- Emphasize the organic, soothing properties of aloe vera and the gentle, natural fragrance of lavender as unique selling points (USP).

This primer's USP lies in its organic, skin-loving ingredients, promising a natural glow and a smooth canvas for makeup application. For commercial use, ensuring compliance with safety standards and highlighting its natural, soothing qualities can attract consumers seeking organic skincare solutions.

Please ensure to seek legal advice or consult with cosmetic experts before commercial production to adhere to safety and regulatory guidelines.

Radiant Green Tea Primer for Natural Beauty

Ingredients:

- Brewed Green Tea (2 tablespoons): Contains antioxidants and anti-inflammatory properties that rejuvenate the skin.
- Aloe Vera Gel (1 teaspoon): Moisturizes and soothes the skin, creating a smooth base for makeup.
- Witch Hazel (1 teaspoon): Acts as a natural astringent, tightening pores and reducing inflammation.
- Jojoba Oil (2-3 drops): Balances skin oil production and provides lightweight hydration.

Description of Ingredients:

- Brewed Green Tea: Rich in polyphenols and catechins, green tea offers antioxidant benefits, protecting the skin from damage and promoting a healthy complexion.
- Aloe Vera Gel: Renowned for its calming and hydrating properties, aloe vera gel soothes the skin and prepares it for makeup application.
- Witch Hazel: A natural toner, witch hazel tightens pores, reduces redness, and helps control excess oil without drying out the skin.
- Jojoba Oil: Resembles the skin's natural oils, making it an excellent moisturizer that doesn't clog pores.

Tools Required:

- Mixing Bowl
- Spoon or Whisk
- Small Airtight Container for Storage

Method:

Homemade Version:

- BREW GREEN TEA: Steep 2 tablespoons of green tea in hot water for a few minutes, then let it cool.
    - Mix Ingredients: In a mixing bowl, combine 1 teaspoon of aloe vera gel, 1 teaspoon of witch hazel, and 2-3 drops of jojoba oil.
    - Add Green Tea: Pour the cooled brewed green tea into the mixture and stir well.
    - Transfer to Container: Pour the mixture into a small airtight container suitable for storage.

Additional Tips:

- Perform a patch test to ensure skin compatibility with the ingredients.
    - Adjust the quantities to suit your skin type; for oily skin, reduce the amount of jojoba oil used.
    - Store the primer in a cool, dry place away from direct sunlight to maintain its potency.

Caution:

- Cease usage if any skin irritation occurs.
    - Avoid contact with eyes; if contact occurs, rinse thoroughly with water.

Commercial Version:

CREATING A COMMERCIAL version requires adherence to safety standards and potential adjustments:

- Certified organic ingredients should be used for commercial production.
    - To extend shelf life, consider adding natural preservatives like vitamin E oil or grapefruit seed extract.
    - Shelf life may range from 6 to 12 months, depending on preservatives used.

• Packaging should prioritize hygiene and product preservation, such as airless pump bottles.

• Emphasize the primer's antioxidant-rich green tea content and the gentle, skin-loving properties of aloe vera and witch hazel as unique selling points (USP).

This primer's USP lies in its organic, antioxidant-rich formulation, promising a natural, radiant complexion. For commercial use, ensuring compliance with safety standards and highlighting its natural, skin-loving qualities can attract consumers seeking organic skincare solutions.

Please seek professional advice or consult cosmetic experts to ensure compliance with safety regulations before commercial production.

Silky Smooth Cornstarch Primer for Perfect Makeup

Ingredients:

- Cornstarch (1 tablespoon): Acts as a natural mattifier, reducing shine and creating a smooth canvas for makeup.
- Aloe Vera Gel (3 tablespoons): Provides hydration and soothes the skin, enhancing the primer's effectiveness.

Description of Ingredients:

- CORNSTARCH: KNOWN for its oil-absorbing properties, cornstarch helps in reducing excess shine on the skin, making it an excellent base for makeup.
- Aloe Vera Gel: Hydrates and calms the skin, ensuring the primer doesn't dry out the skin while providing a smooth texture for makeup application.

Tools Required:

- MIXING BOWL
- Spoon or Whisk
- Small Airtight Container for Storage

Method:

Homemade Version:

MIX INGREDIENTS: IN a mixing bowl, blend 1 tablespoon of cornstarch with 3 tablespoons of aloe vera gel until a smooth paste forms.

Adjust Consistency: If needed, adjust the consistency by adding more aloe vera gel for a thinner texture or more cornstarch for a thicker consistency.

Transfer to Container: Store the mixture in a small airtight container suitable for storage.

Additional Tips:

● PERFORM A PATCH test on a small area of skin to ensure no adverse reactions occur.

    ● Use sparingly; a little goes a long way with this primer.

    ● Store in a cool, dry place away from direct sunlight to maintain its effectiveness.

Caution:

● DISCONTINUE USE if any skin irritation or discomfort arises.

    ● Avoid contact with eyes; if contact occurs, rinse thoroughly with water.

Commercial Version:

CREATING A COMMERCIAL version involves considering safety standards and potential enhancements:

    ● Ensure the use of certified organic ingredients for commercial production.

    ● For extended shelf life, consider adding natural preservatives like vitamin E oil or grapefruit seed extract.

    ● The shelf life may range from 6 to 12 months, depending on preservatives used.

    ● Use hygienic and convenient packaging suitable for dispensing, such as pump bottles or tubes.

    ● Highlight the primer's ability to control shine and create a smooth base for makeup as its unique selling point (USP).

This primer's USP lies in its organic, mattifying properties, ideal for creating a flawless base for makeup application. For commercial use, adhere to safety regulations and emphasize its natural, skin-loving benefits to attract consumers seeking organic skincare solutions.

Prior to commercial production, consult with cosmetic experts to ensure compliance with safety regulations and standards.

Nourishing Moisturizing Oil Primer for Radiant Skin

Ingredients:

- Argan Oil or Rosehip Oil (1 tablespoon): Deeply moisturizes the skin, providing a smooth base for makeup application.
- Shea Butter (1 teaspoon, melted): Offers intense hydration and helps in locking in moisture for a supple complexion.
- Essential Oil (e.g., Frankincense or Geranium) (2-3 drops): Adds a delightful fragrance and may possess additional skin-soothing properties.

Description of Ingredients:

- ARGAN OIL OR ROSEHIP Oil: Rich in fatty acids and antioxidants, these oils deeply hydrate the skin, leaving it soft and smooth.
- Shea Butter: Known for its moisturizing properties, shea butter deeply nourishes the skin and aids in maintaining its moisture balance.
- Essential Oil: Provides a pleasant scent while potentially offering additional skin benefits like soothing or rejuvenating properties.

Tools Required:

- MIXING BOWL
  - Spoon or Whisk
  - Small Airtight Container for Storage

Method:

Homemade Version:

MELT SHEA BUTTER: GENTLY melt 1 teaspoon of shea butter until it becomes liquid.

Mix Ingredients: In a mixing bowl, combine 1 tablespoon of argan oil or rosehip oil with the melted shea butter.

Add Essential Oil: Drop in 2-3 drops of your chosen essential oil and mix thoroughly.

Transfer to Container: Store the mixture in a small airtight container suitable for storage.

Additional Tips:

• PERFORM A PATCH test on a small area of skin to ensure no allergic reactions occur.

• Use a minimal amount of primer, as a little goes a long way.

• Store in a cool, dry place away from direct sunlight to maintain its quality.

Caution:

• DISCONTINUE USE if any skin irritation or discomfort arises.

• Avoid contact with eyes; if contact occurs, rinse thoroughly with water.

Commercial Version:

CREATING A COMMERCIAL version involves considering safety standards and potential enhancements:

• Ensure the use of certified organic ingredients for commercial production.

• Additional stabilizers or natural preservatives like vitamin E oil may be necessary for an extended shelf life.

• Shelf life can vary but may typically range from 6 to 12 months, depending on preservatives used.

• Consider user-friendly packaging, such as pump bottles or tubes, ensuring hygienic and convenient dispensing.

• Highlight the primer's moisturizing properties and potential skin benefits of essential oils as its unique selling point (USP).

The USP of this primer is its organic, deeply moisturizing properties, promising a nourished and hydrated base for makeup. For commercial use, comply with safety regulations and emphasize its natural, skin-loving qualities to appeal to consumers seeking organic skincare solutions.

Consult with cosmetic experts or regulatory authorities to ensure compliance with safety regulations before commercial production.

Refreshing Cucumber Primer for Naturally Glowing Skin

Ingredients:

- Cucumber (½ cucumber, blended or juiced): Provides hydration, soothes the skin, and helps in preparing a smooth basc for makeup.
- Aloe Vera Gel (1 tablespoon): Offers additional hydration and soothes the skin, enhancing the primer's effectiveness.
- Vitamin E Oil (1 teaspoon): Nourishes and moisturizes the skin, promoting a healthy complexion.

Description of Ingredients:

- CUCUMBER: KNOWN for its high water content and soothing properties, cucumber hydrates the skin, reduces puffiness, and primes the skin for makeup application.
- Aloe Vera Gel: Renowned for its calming and hydrating properties, aloe vera gel soothes the skin and enhances the primer's moisturizing effects.
- Vitamin E Oil: Acts as a powerful antioxidant, protecting the skin from damage and deeply moisturizing, resulting in a healthy and radiant complexion.

Tools Required:

- BLENDER OR JUICER
- Mixing Bowl
- Spoon or Whisk
- Small Airtight Container for Storage

Method:

Homemade Version:

PREPARE CUCUMBER: BLEND or juice half a cucumber to extract its liquid content.

Mix Ingredients: In a mixing bowl, combine the cucumber juice or pulp with 1 tablespoon of aloe vera gel.

Add Vitamin E Oil: Add 1 teaspoon of vitamin E oil to the mixture and blend thoroughly.

Transfer to Container: Store the primer mixture in a small airtight container suitable for storage.

Additional Tips:

● PERFORM A PATCH test on a small area of skin to ensure compatibility with the ingredients.

● Keep the primer refrigerated to enhance its refreshing effect when applied to the skin.

● Use a cotton pad or clean hands to apply the primer evenly on the face.

Caution:

● DISCONTINUE USE if any skin irritation or discomfort arises.

● Avoid contact with eyes; if contact occurs, rinse thoroughly with water.

Commercial Version:

CREATING A COMMERCIAL version involves considering safety standards and potential enhancements:

● Use certified organic ingredients for commercial production to appeal to consumers seeking natural skincare solutions.

● Consider adding natural preservatives like grapefruit seed extract to prolong the shelf life, which could range from 6 to 12 months.

- Opt for hygienic and convenient packaging, such as airless pump bottles or squeeze tubes.
- Highlight the primer's refreshing and hydrating properties, emphasizing the use of cucumber and aloe vera as its unique selling point (USP).

The USP of this primer lies in its organic, refreshing properties derived from cucumber and aloe vera, promising a naturally hydrated and glowing skin base for makeup. For commercial use, adhere to safety regulations and emphasize its natural, skin-loving benefits.

Always consult with cosmetic experts or regulatory authorities to ensure compliance with safety regulations before commercial production.

Velvety Rice Powder Primer for a Flawless Base

Ingredients:

- Rice Flour (2 tablespoons): Acts as a natural mattifier, absorbing excess oil and creating a smooth base for makeup.
- Aloe Vera Gel (1 tablespoon): Provides hydration and soothes the skin, enhancing the primer's effectiveness.
- Jojoba Oil (½ teaspoon): Balances skin oil production and offers lightweight hydration.
- Lavender Essential Oil (2-3 drops): Adds a pleasant fragrance and may possess calming properties for the skin.

Description of Ingredients:

- RICE FLOUR: KNOWN for its oil-absorbing properties, rice flour helps in reducing shine on the skin, making it an excellent base for makeup.
- Aloe Vera Gel: Hydrates and calms the skin, ensuring the primer doesn't dry out the skin while providing a smooth texture for makeup application.
- Jojoba Oil: Resembles the skin's natural oils, making it an excellent moisturizer that doesn't clog pores.
- Lavender Essential Oil: Provides a delightful scent and may have additional soothing effects on the skin.

Tools Required:

- MIXING BOWL
- Spoon or Whisk
- Small Airtight Container for Storage

Method:

Homemade Version:

MIX INGREDIENTS: IN a mixing bowl, combine 2 tablespoons of rice flour with 1 tablespoon of aloe vera gel.

Add Jojoba Oil: Incorporate ½ teaspoon of jojoba oil into the mixture and blend thoroughly.

Drop Essential Oil: Add 2-3 drops of lavender essential oil for a pleasant fragrance and mix well.

Store: Transfer the primer mixture into a small airtight container suitable for storage.

Additional Tips:

● PERFORM A PATCH test on a small area of skin to ensure no allergic reactions occur.

● Use a small amount of primer for application, as a little goes a long way.

● Store the primer in a cool, dry place away from direct sunlight to maintain its quality.

Caution:

● DISCONTINUE USE if any skin irritation or discomfort arises.

● Avoid contact with eyes; if contact occurs, rinse thoroughly with water.

Commercial Version:

CREATING A COMMERCIAL version involves considering safety standards and potential enhancements:

● Utilize certified organic ingredients for commercial production.

● Consider adding natural preservatives like vitamin E oil to prolong the shelf life, which could range from 6 to 12 months.

● Opt for convenient and hygienic packaging, such as airless pump bottles or jars with spatulas for application.

- Emphasize the primer's ability to control shine and create a smooth, matte base for makeup as its unique selling point (USP).

The USP of this primer lies in its organic, mattifying properties derived from rice flour and aloe vera, promising a flawless base for makeup application. For commercial use, comply with safety regulations and highlight its natural, skin-loving benefits.

Always consult with cosmetic experts or regulatory authorities to ensure compliance with safety regulations before commercial production.

Luxurious Shea Butter Primer for Hydrated Skin

Ingredients:

- Shea Butter (1 tablespoon, melted): Offers intense hydration and helps in creating a smooth base for makeup.
- Coconut Oil (1 teaspoon): Provides additional moisturization and aids in maintaining skin elasticity.
- Aloe Vera Gel (1 teaspoon): Soothes the skin and enhances the primer's hydrating properties.
- Vitamin E Oil (2-3 drops): Nourishes and protects the skin, promoting a healthy complexion.

Description of Ingredients:

- SHEA BUTTER: RENOWNED for its moisturizing properties, shea butter deeply nourishes the skin and aids in maintaining its moisture balance.
- Coconut Oil: Contains fatty acids that moisturize and protect the skin, leaving it soft and supple.
- Aloe Vera Gel: Known for its calming and hydrating properties, aloe vera gel soothes the skin and enhances the primer's effectiveness.
- Vitamin E Oil: Acts as a potent antioxidant, protecting the skin from damage and deeply moisturizing for a healthy glow.

Tools Required:

- MIXING BOWL
- Spoon or Whisk
- Small Airtight Container for Storage

Method:

Homemade Version:

MELT SHEA BUTTER: GENTLY melt 1 tablespoon of shea butter until it becomes liquid.

Mix Ingredients: In a mixing bowl, combine the melted shea butter with 1 teaspoon of coconut oil and 1 teaspoon of aloe vera gel.

Add Vitamin E Oil: Incorporate 2-3 drops of vitamin E oil into the mixture and blend thoroughly.

Store: Transfer the primer mixture into a small airtight container suitable for storage.

Additional Tips:

● CONDUCT A PATCH test on a small area of skin to ensure no adverse reactions occur.

● Use a small amount of primer for application; a little goes a long way.

● Store the primer in a cool, dry place away from direct sunlight to maintain its quality.

Caution:

● DISCONTINUE USE if any skin irritation or discomfort arises.

● Avoid contact with eyes; if contact occurs, rinse thoroughly with water.

Commercial Version:

CREATING A COMMERCIAL version involves considering safety standards and potential enhancements:

● Use certified organic ingredients for commercial production.

● Consider adding natural preservatives like grapefruit seed extract to extend the shelf life, which could range from 6 to 12 months.

● Opt for hygienic and practical packaging, such as airless pump bottles or jars with spatulas for easy application.

● Highlight the primer's luxurious hydrating properties derived from shea butter as its unique selling point (USP).

The USP of this primer lies in its organic, luxurious hydration offered by shea butter, promising a nourished and smooth base for makeup. For commercial use, ensure compliance with safety regulations and emphasize its natural, skin-loving benefits.

Consult with cosmetic experts or regulatory authorities to ensure compliance with safety regulations before commercial production.

Soothing Oatmeal Primer for a Natural Glow

Ingredients:

- Oatmeal (2 tablespoons, finely ground): Acts as a gentle exfoliant, soothes the skin, and helps in creating a smooth base for makeup.
- Aloe Vera Gel (1 tablespoon): Provides hydration and calms the skin, enhancing the primer's effectiveness.
- Coconut Oil (½ teaspoon): Adds moisturization and aids in maintaining skin softness.

Description of Ingredients:

- OATMEAL: KNOWN FOR its calming properties, finely ground oatmeal acts as a gentle exfoliant, smoothing the skin's surface and creating an ideal base for makeup.
- Aloe Vera Gel: Hydrates and soothes the skin, ensuring the primer doesn't dry out the skin while providing a smooth texture for makeup application.
- Coconut Oil: Contains fatty acids that moisturize and protect the skin, leaving it soft and supple.

Tools Required:

- BLENDER OR FOOD Processor (for grinding oatmeal)
- Mixing Bowl
- Spoon or Whisk
- Small Airtight Container for Storage

Method:

Homemade Version:

GRIND OATMEAL: USE a blender or food processor to finely grind 2 tablespoons of oatmeal.

Mix Ingredients: In a mixing bowl, combine the ground oatmeal with 1 tablespoon of aloe vera gel and ½ teaspoon of coconut oil.

Blend Thoroughly: Mix the ingredients well until a smooth paste-like consistency is achieved.

Store: Transfer the primer mixture into a small airtight container suitable for storage.

Additional Tips:

● PERFORM A PATCH test on a small area of skin to ensure no allergic reactions occur.

● Use a small amount of primer for application; a little goes a long way.

● Store the primer in a cool, dry place away from direct sunlight to maintain its quality.

Caution:

● DISCONTINUE USE if any skin irritation or discomfort arises.

● Avoid contact with eyes; if contact occurs, rinse thoroughly with water.

Commercial Version:

CREATING A COMMERCIAL version involves considering safety standards and potential enhancements:

● Use certified organic ingredients for commercial production to appeal to consumers seeking natural skincare solutions.

● Consider adding natural preservatives like vitamin E oil to prolong the shelf life, which could range from 6 to 12 months.

● Opt for convenient and hygienic packaging, such as airless pump bottles or jars with spatulas for easy application.

● Emphasize the primer's soothing and gentle exfoliating properties derived from oatmeal as its unique selling point (USP).

The USP of this primer lies in its organic, soothing properties derived from oatmeal, promising a calm and smooth base for makeup. For commercial use, comply with safety regulations and highlight its natural, skin-loving benefits.

Always consult with cosmetic experts or regulatory authorities to ensure compliance with safety regulations before commercial production.

Silky Almond Oil Primer for a Perfect Makeup Base

Ingredients:

- Almond Oil (1 tablespoon): Nourishes and softens the skin, creating a smooth canvas for makeup.
- Aloe Vera Gel (1 tablespoon): Provides hydration and soothes the skin, enhancing the primer's effectiveness.
- Beeswax (½ teaspoon, grated): Adds a light barrier and helps in maintaining the primer's consistency.

Description of Ingredients:

- ALMOND OIL: RICH in vitamins and fatty acids, almond oil deeply moisturizes the skin, leaving it soft and supple while creating an ideal base for makeup.
- Aloe Vera Gel: Renowned for its calming and hydrating properties, aloe vera gel soothes the skin and enhances the primer's moisturizing effects.
- Beeswax: Acts as a natural emulsifier and thickening agent, helping to maintain the primer's texture and providing a light barrier on the skin.

Tools Required:

- MIXING BOWL
- Double Boiler or Microwave-Safe Bowl
- Spoon or Whisk
- Small Airtight Container for Storage

Method:

Homemade Version:

MELT BEESWAX: USE A double boiler or microwave-safe bowl to gently melt ½ teaspoon of grated beeswax until it liquefies.

Combine Ingredients: In a mixing bowl, mix together 1 tablespoon of almond oil, 1 tablespoon of aloe vera gel, and the melted beeswax.

Blend Thoroughly: Stir the ingredients well until they are thoroughly combined and form a smooth mixture.

Store: Transfer the primer mixture into a small airtight container suitable for storage.

Additional Tips:

● PERFORM A PATCH test on a small area of skin to ensure compatibility with the ingredients.

● Use a small amount of primer for application, as a little goes a long way.

● Store the primer in a cool, dry place away from direct sunlight to maintain its quality.

Caution:

● DISCONTINUE USE if any skin irritation or discomfort arises.

● Avoid contact with eyes; if contact occurs, rinse thoroughly with water.

Commercial Version:

CREATING A COMMERCIAL version involves considering safety standards and potential enhancements:

● Utilize certified organic ingredients for commercial production to appeal to consumers seeking natural skincare solutions.

● Consider adding natural preservatives like grapefruit seed extract to extend the shelf life, which could range from 6 to 12 months.

● Opt for hygienic and practical packaging, such as airless pump bottles or jars with spatulas for easy application.

● Highlight the primer's nourishing and moisturizing properties derived from almond oil as its unique selling point (USP).

The USP of this primer lies in its organic, nourishing properties derived from almond oil, promising a smooth and hydrated base for makeup. For commercial use, ensure compliance with safety regulations and emphasize its natural, skin-loving benefits.

Always consult with cosmetic experts or regulatory authorities to ensure compliance with safety regulations before commercial production.

Organic Mineral Powder Foundation Recipe

Ingredients:

- Arrowroot Powder (1/4 cup): A natural root starch that helps in absorbing excess oils.
- Cocoa Powder (2 tablespoons): Provides color and helps in achieving the desired shade.
- Bentonite Clay (1 tablespoon): Known for its detoxifying properties, it aids in skin health.
- Ground Cinnamon (1/2 teaspoon): Adds warmth and tone to the foundation.
- Ground Nutmeg (1/4 teaspoon): Adds a subtle hue and offers skin benefits.

Tools Required:

- MIXING BOWL
- Measuring spoons
- Small sieve or sifter
- Airtight container for storage

Method:

1. Homemade Version:

- MEASURE INGREDIENTS: Take the arrowroot powder, cocoa powder, bentonite clay, ground cinnamon, and ground nutmeg.
- Mix Thoroughly: In a mixing bowl, combine all the ingredients well. Use a sieve or sifter to ensure a smooth and even texture.
- Test Shade: Test the shade on your skin to check if it matches your tone. Adjust the quantities of cocoa powder or cinnamon to achieve the desired color.
- Storage: Store the foundation in an airtight container away from moisture and direct sunlight.

Additional Tips:

● *Customize Shade:* Adjust the quantities of cocoa powder or cinnamon to match your skin tone perfectly.

● *Essential Oils:* Add a few drops of organic essential oil for added skincare benefits and fragrance. Lavender or tea tree oil are good options.

Caution:

● PATCH TEST THE FOUNDATION on a small area of your skin before applying it to the face to ensure no adverse reactions occur.

Commercial Version:

MAKING A COMMERCIAL version of this foundation could be a great idea! To scale up and enhance the product for commercial use:

● Additional Ingredients: Consider adding organic rice flour for a smoother texture and enhanced coverage (1/4 cup).

● Method Changes: Use specialized machinery for thorough mixing and to maintain consistency in large batches.

● Packaging Tips: Opt for eco-friendly, branded packaging that highlights its organic nature. Seal it properly to prevent moisture ingress.

● Shelf Life: The shelf life for the commercial version can be around 6-12 months if stored in ideal conditions.

Unique Selling Proposition (USP):

THIS ORGANIC MINERAL powder foundation offers a natural alternative to conventional makeup. Its blend of organic ingredients ensures a healthier choice for your skin, providing coverage while promoting skin wellness.

Crafting organic cosmetics requires precision and care, and creating a commercial version demands compliance with regulations and testing. Always ensure legal compliance and safety standards for commercial production.

Organic Shea Butter Foundation Recipe

Ingredients:

- Shea Butter (2 tablespoons): Moisturizes the skin and provides a creamy base for the foundation.
- Jojoba Oil (1 tablespoon): Helps balance skin's natural oils and aids in blending.
- Zinc Oxide (1 teaspoon): Offers natural sun protection and coverage.
- Cocoa Powder (1/2 teaspoon): Adds color and tone to match various skin shades.

Tools Required:

- MIXING BOWL
  - Double boiler or microwave
  - Measuring spoons
  - Small container for storage

Method:

1. Homemade Version:

- MELT SHEA BUTTER: Use a double boiler or microwave to melt the shea butter until it becomes liquid.
  - Combine Ingredients: In a mixing bowl, blend the melted shea butter with jojoba oil, zinc oxide, and cocoa powder until it forms a smooth mixture.
  - Test & Adjust: Apply a small amount to your skin to check the shade and coverage. Adjust the cocoa powder quantity for your desired shade.
  - Storage: Transfer the foundation into a small, clean container for storage. Keep it in a cool, dry place.

Additional Tips:

- *Customize Shade & Coverage:* Adjust the cocoa powder quantity for lighter or darker shades. Add more zinc oxide for increased coverage.
- *Essential Oils:* Consider adding a few drops of organic essential oils for added fragrance and skin benefits.

Caution:

- PATCH TEST THE FOUNDATION on a small area of your skin before applying it to the face to ensure no adverse reactions occur.

Commercial Version:

CREATING A COMMERCIAL version of this foundation could be a good idea! To make it suitable for commercial use:

- Additional Ingredients: Include organic arrowroot powder (1 teaspoon) for a smoother finish and enhanced coverage.
- Method Changes: Use precise measurements and professional equipment for consistency in larger batches.
- Packaging Tips: Opt for elegant, eco-friendly packaging that highlights its organic nature. Ensure proper sealing for longer shelf life and product integrity.
- Shelf Life: The shelf life for the commercial version can be around 6-12 months when stored in ideal conditions.

Unique Selling Proposition (USP):

THIS ORGANIC SHEA BUTTER Foundation offers natural coverage while nourishing the skin with its blend of organic ingredients. It provides a smooth, moisturizing base and is suitable for various skin types, showcasing its skincare benefits alongside coverage.

Creating cosmetics for commercial use involves following safety standards, compliance with regulations, and ensuring accurate labeling. Always ensure legal compliance and safety standards for commercial production.

Organic Arrowroot Powder Foundation Recipe

Ingredients:

- Arrowroot Powder (1/4 cup): This natural starch helps absorb oils and provides a smooth texture.
- Cocoa Powder (2 tablespoons): Adds color and helps match different skin tones organically.
- Ground Cinnamon (1/2 teaspoon): Provides warmth and contributes to the foundation's shade.
- Zinc Oxide (1 tablespoon): Offers natural sun protection and additional coverage.

Tools Required:

- MIXING BOWL
  - Measuring spoons
  - Small sieve or sifter
  - Airtight container for storage

Method:

1. Homemade Version:

- COMBINE INGREDIENTS: In a mixing bowl, blend arrowroot powder, cocoa powder, ground cinnamon, and zinc oxide thoroughly.
- Sift for Consistency: Use a small sieve or sifter to ensure an even texture and eliminate any lumps.
- Test & Adjust: Test the shade by applying a small amount to your skin. Adjust cocoa powder for lighter or darker shades.
- Storage: Store the foundation in an airtight container away from moisture and direct sunlight.

Additional Tips:

● *Customize Shade & Coverage:* Adjust cocoa powder for desired shades. Add more zinc oxide for increased coverage or sun protection.

● *Essential Oils:* Consider adding a drop of organic essential oil for fragrance and added skincare benefits.

Caution:

● PERFORM A PATCH test on a small area of your skin before applying the foundation to ensure no adverse reactions occur.

Commercial Version:

CREATING A COMMERCIAL version of this foundation could be a good idea! For a commercial-scale preparation, consider:

● Additional Ingredients: Include organic rice flour (1/4 cup) for a smoother texture and enhanced coverage.

● Method Changes: Use professional mixing equipment for consistency in larger batches.

● Packaging Tips: Opt for eco-friendly, labeled packaging that emphasizes its organic nature. Ensure proper sealing for longer shelf life.

● Shelf Life: The shelf life for the commercial version can be around 6-12 months if stored properly.

Unique Selling Proposition (USP):

THIS ORGANIC ARROWROOT Powder Foundation offers a natural alternative to conventional makeup. Its blend of organic ingredients ensures a healthier choice for your skin, providing coverage while promoting skin wellness.

Crafting organic cosmetics requires attention to detail, safety considerations, and complying with regulations for commercial production. Always ensure legal compliance and safety standards.

Natural Radiance Organic Cornstarch Foundation Recipe

Ingredients:

- Cornstarch (1/4 cup): A natural absorbent that provides a smooth texture to the foundation.
- Cocoa Powder (1 tablespoon): Adds color and helps match various skin tones organically.
- Ground Cinnamon (1/2 teaspoon): Provides warmth and contributes to the foundation's shade.
- Zinc Oxide (1 tablespoon): Offers natural sun protection and additional coverage.

Tools Required:

- MIXING BOWL
  - Measuring spoons
  - Small sieve or sifter
  - Airtight container for storage

Method:

1. Homemade Version:

- BLEND INGREDIENTS: In a mixing bowl, combine cornstarch, cocoa powder, ground cinnamon, and zinc oxide thoroughly.
  - Sieve for Consistency: Use a small sieve or sifter to ensure a lump-free, smooth texture.
  - Adjust Shade & Test: Test the shade by applying a small amount to your skin. Adjust cocoa powder for lighter or darker shades as desired.
  - Storage: Store the foundation in an airtight container away from moisture and direct sunlight.

Additional Tips:

● *Customize Shade & Coverage:* Adjust cocoa powder quantities for different shades. Increase zinc oxide for more coverage or sun protection.

● *Essential Oils:* Consider adding a drop of organic essential oil for a pleasant scent and added skincare benefits.

Caution:

● ALWAYS PERFORM A patch test on a small area of your skin before applying the foundation to ensure no adverse reactions occur.

Commercial Version:

DEVELOPING A COMMERCIAL version of this foundation might be a good idea! For a commercial-scale preparation, consider:

● Additional Ingredients: Incorporate organic rice flour (1/4 cup) for a smoother texture and enhanced coverage.

● Method Changes: Use professional-grade equipment for consistency in larger batches.

● Packaging Tips: Opt for eco-friendly, labeled packaging that emphasizes its organic nature. Ensure proper sealing for a longer shelf life.

● Shelf Life: The shelf life for the commercial version can be around 6-12 months if stored correctly.

Unique Selling Proposition (USP):

THIS ORGANIC CORNSTARCH Foundation offers a natural and gentle alternative to traditional makeup. It not only provides coverage but also promotes skin health through its organic ingredients, offering a more radiant look while caring for the skin.

Crafting organic cosmetics for commercial use requires adherence to safety regulations, meticulous testing, and compliance with labeling laws. Always ensure legal compliance and safety standards.

Organic Nourish & Glow: Homemade Liquid Foundation with Oils

Ingredients:

- Jojoba Oil (2 tablespoons): Mimics the skin's natural oils, providing hydration and aiding in blending.
- Argan Oil (1 tablespoon): Rich in antioxidants and Vitamin E, it nourishes the skin and helps in achieving a smooth texture.
- Shea Butter (1 tablespoon): Moisturizes and softens the skin, providing a creamy base for the foundation.
- Zinc Oxide (1 teaspoon): Offers natural sun protection and additional coverage.
- Arrowroot Powder (1 teaspoon): Acts as a thickening agent and provides a matte finish.

Tools Required:

- MIXING BOWL
  - Double boiler or microwave
  - Measuring spoons
  - Small container for storage

Method:

1. Homemade Version:

- MELT INGREDIENTS: Use a double boiler or microwave to melt the shea butter until it becomes liquid. Combine it with jojoba oil and argan oil in a mixing bowl.
- Add Powders: Mix in zinc oxide and arrowroot powder gradually while stirring continuously until a smooth consistency is achieved.
- Test & Adjust: Apply a small amount to your skin to test the shade and coverage. Adjust the powder quantities for desired shades or coverage.

- Storage: Transfer the foundation into a clean, small container for storage. Keep it in a cool, dry place away from direct sunlight.

Additional Tips:

- *Customize Shade & Texture:* Adjust the powder quantities for lighter or darker shades. Increase arrowroot powder for a matte finish.
- *Essential Oils:* Consider adding a drop of organic essential oil for a pleasant scent and added skincare benefits.

Caution:

- ALWAYS CONDUCT A patch test on a small area of your skin before applying the foundation to ensure no adverse reactions occur.

Commercial Version:

CREATING A COMMERCIAL version of this foundation could be beneficial! To modify it for commercial use:

- Additional Ingredients: Include organic rice flour (1 teaspoon) for a smoother texture and enhanced coverage.
- Method Changes: Use professional-grade equipment for consistency in larger batches.
- Packaging Tips: Opt for eco-friendly, labeled packaging that highlights its organic nature. Ensure proper sealing for a longer shelf life.
- Shelf Life: The shelf life for the commercial version can be around 6-12 months if stored correctly.

Unique Selling Proposition (USP):

THIS ORGANIC LIQUID Foundation with Oils offers a nourishing, hydrating, and protective blend of ingredients. It not only provides coverage but also cares for the skin, offering a natural radiance and nourishment, making it an ideal choice for those seeking both coverage and skincare benefits.

Creating cosmetics for commercial use requires careful adherence to safety regulations, rigorous testing, and compliance with labeling laws. Always ensure legal compliance and safety standards.

Organic Radiance Blend: Homemade Rice Flour Foundation

Ingredients:

- Rice Flour (1/4 cup): Known for its gentle exfoliating properties, it helps create a smooth base and offers a natural matte finish.
- Shea Butter (1 tablespoon): Provides moisture and helps in achieving a creamy texture for the foundation.
- Jojoba Oil (1 tablespoon): Balances natural oils, hydrates the skin, and aids in blending.
- Zinc Oxide (1 teaspoon): Provides natural sun protection and additional coverage.

Tools Required:

- MIXING BOWL
  - Double boiler or microwave
  - Measuring spoons
  - Small container for storage

Method:

1. Homemade Version:

- MELT INGREDIENTS: Use a double boiler or microwave to melt the shea butter until it becomes liquid. Combine it with jojoba oil in a mixing bowl.
- Add Rice Flour & Zinc Oxide: Gradually mix in the rice flour and zinc oxide, stirring continuously until a smooth consistency is achieved.
- Test & Adjust: Apply a small amount to your skin to test the shade and coverage. Adjust rice flour or zinc oxide quantities for desired shades or coverage.
- Storage: Transfer the foundation into a clean, small container for storage. Keep it in a cool, dry place away from direct sunlight.

Additional Tips:

• *Customize Shade & Coverage:* Adjust rice flour or zinc oxide quantities for lighter or darker shades. Increase rice flour for a matte finish.

• *Essential Oils:* Consider adding a drop of organic essential oil for a pleasant scent and added skincare benefits.

Caution:

• ALWAYS PERFORM A patch test on a small area of your skin before applying the foundation to ensure no adverse reactions occur.

Commercial Version:

DEVELOPING A COMMERCIAL version of this foundation might be beneficial! To modify it for commercial use:

• Additional Ingredients: Include organic arrowroot powder (1 teaspoon) for a smoother texture and enhanced coverage.

• Method Changes: Use professional-grade equipment for consistency in larger batches.

• Packaging Tips: Opt for eco-friendly, labeled packaging that highlights its organic nature. Ensure proper sealing for a longer shelf life.

• Shelf Life: The shelf life for the commercial version can be around 6-12 months if stored correctly.

Unique Selling Proposition (USP):

THIS ORGANIC RICE FLOUR Foundation offers a blend of gentle exfoliation, natural coverage, and moisturization. It not only evens out the skin tone but also nurtures the skin, promoting a radiant and healthy complexion.

Crafting cosmetics for commercial use requires adherence to safety regulations, meticulous testing, and compliance with labeling laws. Always ensure legal compliance and safety standards.

Natural Glow: Homemade Beeswax Foundation

Ingredients:

- Beeswax (2 tablespoons): Acts as a natural thickening agent, providing structure and stability to the foundation.
- Coconut Oil (1 tablespoon): Hydrates and moisturizes the skin while aiding in blending and creating a smooth texture.
- Shea Butter (1 tablespoon): Offers moisture and helps in achieving a creamy consistency for the foundation.
- Arrowroot Powder (1 teaspoon): Helps in mattifying the foundation and offering a smoother finish.

Tools Required:

- DOUBLE BOILER OR microwave
- Mixing bowl
- Measuring spoons
- Small container for storage

Method:

1. Homemade Version:

- MELT INGREDIENTS: Use a double boiler or microwave to melt the beeswax until it becomes liquid. Add coconut oil and shea butter, allowing them to melt together.
- Incorporate Arrowroot Powder: Gradually add arrowroot powder while stirring continuously to ensure even mixing and to avoid lumps.
- Test & Adjust: Apply a small amount to your skin to test the shade and coverage. Adjust arrowroot powder for a matte finish or to match desired shades.
- Storage: Transfer the foundation into a clean, small container for storage. Store it in a cool, dry place away from direct sunlight.

Additional Tips:

- *Customize Texture & Finish:* Adjust arrowroot powder quantities for a matte finish. Increase coconut oil for a more hydrating foundation.
- *Essential Oils:* Consider adding a drop of organic essential oil for a pleasant scent and added skincare benefits.

Caution:

- PERFORM A PATCH test on a small area of your skin before applying the foundation to ensure no adverse reactions occur.

Commercial Version:

CREATING A COMMERCIAL version of this foundation could be advantageous! To modify it for commercial use:

- Additional Ingredients: Include organic jojoba oil (1 tablespoon) for added skin benefits and a smoother texture.
- Method Changes: Use professional-grade equipment for consistency in larger batches.
- Packaging Tips: Opt for eco-friendly, labeled packaging that emphasizes its organic nature. Ensure proper sealing for a longer shelf life.
- Shelf Life: The shelf life for the commercial version can be around 6-12 months if stored correctly.

Unique Selling Proposition (USP):

THIS ORGANIC BEESWAX Foundation offers a blend of natural ingredients that provide structure, hydration, and a smooth finish. It not only acts as a foundation but also nourishes the skin, promoting a healthy glow.

Crafting cosmetics for commercial use requires compliance with safety regulations, meticulous testing, and adherence to labeling laws. Always ensure legal compliance and safety standards.

Natural Radiance: Homemade Aloe Vera Gel Foundation

Ingredients:

● Aloe Vera Gel (2 tablespoons): Provides hydration and soothes the skin, acting as a base for the foundation.

● Coconut Oil (1 tablespoon): Offers moisture and helps in achieving a smooth texture for the foundation.

● Shea Butter (1 tablespoon): Provides moisture and helps in achieving a creamy consistency for the foundation.

● Arrowroot Powder (1 teaspoon): Acts as a thickening agent and provides a matte finish.

Tools Required:

● DOUBLE BOILER OR microwave
  ● Mixing bowl
  ● Measuring spoons
  ● Small container for storage

Method:

1. Homemade Version:

● MELT INGREDIENTS: Use a double boiler or microwave to melt the shea butter until it becomes liquid. Add coconut oil to the melted shea butter.

● Combine with Aloe Vera Gel: Mix the melted mixture with aloe vera gel in a mixing bowl until well incorporated.

● Incorporate Arrowroot Powder: Gradually add arrowroot powder while stirring continuously to ensure an even mixture and to avoid lumps.

● Test & Adjust: Apply a small amount to your skin to test the shade and coverage. Adjust arrowroot powder for a matte finish or to match desired shades.

- Storage: Transfer the foundation into a clean, small container for storage. Keep it in a cool, dry place away from direct sunlight.

Additional Tips:

- *Customize Texture & Finish:* Adjust arrowroot powder quantities for a matte finish. Increase aloe vera gel for a more hydrating foundation.
- *Essential Oils:* Consider adding a drop of organic essential oil for a pleasant scent and added skincare benefits.

Caution:

- PERFORM A PATCH test on a small area of your skin before applying the foundation to ensure no adverse reactions occur.

Commercial Version:

DEVELOPING A COMMERCIAL version of this foundation might be beneficial! To modify it for commercial use:

- Additional Ingredients: Include organic jojoba oil (1 tablespoon) for added skin benefits and a smoother texture.
- Method Changes: Use professional-grade equipment for consistency in larger batches.
- Packaging Tips: Opt for eco-friendly, labeled packaging that emphasizes its organic nature. Ensure proper sealing for a longer shelf life.
- Shelf Life: The shelf life for the commercial version can be around 6-12 months if stored correctly.

Unique Selling Proposition (USP):

THIS ORGANIC ALOE VERA Gel Foundation offers a blend of natural ingredients that provide hydration, moisture, and a smooth finish. It not only acts as a foundation but also nurtures the skin, promoting a healthy and radiant complexion.

Crafting cosmetics for commercial use requires compliance with safety regulations, meticulous testing, and adherence to labeling laws. Always ensure legal compliance and safety standards.

Pure Radiance: Homemade Kaolin Clay Foundation

Ingredients:

- Kaolin Clay (2 tablespoons): Known for its gentle cleansing and oil-absorbing properties, it provides a smooth texture and a natural matte finish.
- Shea Butter (1 tablespoon): Offers moisture and helps in achieving a creamy consistency for the foundation.
- Jojoba Oil (1 tablespoon): Balances natural oils, hydrates the skin, and aids in blending.
- Zinc Oxide (1 teaspoon): Provides natural sun protection and additional coverage.

Tools Required:

- DOUBLE BOILER OR microwave
- Mixing bowl
- Measuring spoons
- Small container for storage

Method:

1. Homemade Version:

- MELT INGREDIENTS: Use a double boiler or microwave to melt the shea butter until it becomes liquid. Combine it with jojoba oil in a mixing bowl.
- Mix in Kaolin Clay: Gradually add kaolin clay while stirring continuously to ensure an even mixture.
- Incorporate Zinc Oxide: Mix in zinc oxide gradually, ensuring it is evenly distributed for added coverage and sun protection.

- Test & Adjust: Apply a small amount to your skin to test the shade and coverage. Adjust kaolin clay or zinc oxide quantities for desired shades or coverage.
- Storage: Transfer the foundation into a clean, small container for storage. Keep it in a cool, dry place away from direct sunlight.

Additional Tips:

- *Customize Texture & Finish:* Adjust kaolin clay quantities for a matte finish. Increase jojoba oil for a more hydrating foundation.
- *Essential Oils:* Consider adding a drop of organic essential oil for a pleasant scent and added skincare benefits.

Caution:

- PERFORM A PATCH test on a small area of your skin before applying the foundation to ensure no adverse reactions occur.

Commercial Version:

DEVELOPING A COMMERCIAL version of this foundation might be beneficial! To modify it for commercial use:

- Additional Ingredients: Include organic arrowroot powder (1 teaspoon) for a smoother texture and enhanced coverage.
- Method Changes: Use professional-grade equipment for consistency in larger batches.
- Packaging Tips: Opt for eco-friendly, labeled packaging that emphasizes its organic nature. Ensure proper sealing for a longer shelf life.
- Shelf Life: The shelf life for the commercial version can be around 6-12 months if stored correctly.

Unique Selling Proposition (USP):

THIS ORGANIC KAOLIN Clay Foundation offers a blend of natural ingredients that provide oil-absorption, coverage, and hydration. It not only acts as a foundation but also nurtures the skin, promoting a healthy and even complexion.

Crafting cosmetics for commercial use requires compliance with safety regulations, meticulous testing, and adherence to labeling laws. Always ensure legal compliance and safety standards.

Natural Glow: Homemade Tapioca Flour Foundation

Ingredients:

- Tapioca Flour (2 tablespoons): Acts as a thickening agent, providing a smooth texture and natural coverage to the foundation.
- Shea Butter (1 tablespoon): Offers moisture and helps in achieving a creamy consistency for the foundation.
- Coconut Oil (1 tablespoon): Hydrates and nourishes the skin while aiding in blending.
- Zinc Oxide (1 teaspoon): Provides natural sun protection and additional coverage.

Tools Required:

- DOUBLE BOILER OR microwave
- Mixing bowl
- Measuring spoons
- Small container for storage

Method:

1. Homemade Version:

- MELT INGREDIENTS: Use a double boiler or microwave to melt the shea butter until it becomes liquid. Combine it with coconut oil in a mixing bowl.
- Incorporate Tapioca Flour: Gradually add tapioca flour while stirring continuously to ensure an even mixture.
- Add Zinc Oxide: Mix in zinc oxide gradually, ensuring it is evenly distributed for added coverage and sun protection.
- Test & Adjust: Apply a small amount to your skin to test the shade and coverage. Adjust tapioca flour or zinc oxide quantities for desired shades or coverage.

• Storage: Transfer the foundation into a clean, small container for storage. Keep it in a cool, dry place away from direct sunlight.

Additional Tips:

• *Customize Texture & Finish:* Adjust tapioca flour quantities for a matte finish. Increase coconut oil for a more hydrating foundation.

• *Essential Oils:* Consider adding a drop of organic essential oil for a pleasant scent and added skincare benefits.

Caution:

• PERFORM A PATCH test on a small area of your skin before applying the foundation to ensure no adverse reactions occur.

Commercial Version:

DEVELOPING A COMMERCIAL version of this foundation might be advantageous! To modify it for commercial use:

• Additional Ingredients: Include organic arrowroot powder (1 teaspoon) for a smoother texture and enhanced coverage.

• Method Changes: Use professional-grade equipment for consistency in larger batches.

• Packaging Tips: Opt for eco-friendly, labeled packaging that emphasizes its organic nature. Ensure proper sealing for a longer shelf life.

• Shelf Life: The shelf life for the commercial version can be around 6-12 months if stored correctly.

Unique Selling Proposition (USP):

THIS ORGANIC TAPIOCA Flour Foundation offers a blend of natural ingredients that provide a smooth texture, coverage, and hydration. It not only acts as a foundation but also nurtures the skin, promoting a healthy and radiant complexion.

Crafting cosmetics for commercial use requires compliance with safety regulations, meticulous testing, and adherence to labeling laws. Always ensure legal compliance and safety standards.

Natural Radiance: Homemade Sunflower Seed Oil and Cocoa Powder Foundation

Ingredients:

- Sunflower Seed Oil (2 tablespoons): Acts as a base, providing moisture and aiding in blending the foundation.
- Cocoa Powder (2 teaspoons): Provides color pigmentation and coverage, offering a natural tint to the foundation.
- Arrowroot Powder (1 teaspoon): Acts as a thickening agent and provides a smooth, matte finish.
- Shea Butter (1 tablespoon): Offers moisture and helps in achieving a creamy consistency for the foundation.

Tools Required:

- DOUBLE BOILER OR microwave
- Mixing bowl
- Measuring spoons
- Small container for storage

Method:

1. Homemade Version:

- MELT INGREDIENTS: Use a double boiler or microwave to melt the shea butter until it becomes liquid. Combine it with sunflower seed oil in a mixing bowl.
- Incorporate Cocoa Powder: Gradually add cocoa powder while stirring continuously to ensure an even mixture and desired shade.
- Mix in Arrowroot Powder: Gradually add arrowroot powder while stirring continuously to achieve desired consistency and a matte finish.
- Test & Adjust: Apply a small amount to your skin to test the shade and coverage. Adjust cocoa powder or arrowroot powder quantities for desired shades or coverage.

- Storage: Transfer the foundation into a clean, small container for storage. Keep it in a cool, dry place away from direct sunlight.

Additional Tips:

- *Customize Shade & Texture:* Adjust cocoa powder quantities for lighter or darker shades. Increase arrowroot powder for a matte finish.
- *Essential Oils:* Consider adding a drop of organic essential oil for a pleasant scent and added skincare benefits.

Caution:

- ALWAYS PERFORM A patch test on a small area of your skin before applying the foundation to ensure no adverse reactions occur.

Commercial Version:

DEVELOPING A COMMERCIAL version of this foundation might be beneficial! To modify it for commercial use:

- Additional Ingredients: Include organic jojoba oil (1 tablespoon) for added skincare benefits and a smoother texture.
- Method Changes: Use professional-grade equipment for consistency in larger batches.
- Packaging Tips: Opt for eco-friendly, labeled packaging that emphasizes its organic nature. Ensure proper sealing for a longer shelf life.
- Shelf Life: The shelf life for the commercial version can be around 6-12 months if stored correctly.

Unique Selling Proposition (USP):

THIS ORGANIC SUNFLOWER Seed Oil and Cocoa Powder Foundation offer a natural tint, coverage, and hydration. It provides a healthy glow and skincare benefits, catering to those seeking both coverage and nourishment.

Crafting cosmetics for commercial use requires compliance with safety regulations, meticulous testing, and adherence to labeling laws. Always ensure legal compliance and safety standards.

Ethereal Glow: Homemade Frankincense Essential Oil Foundation

Ingredients:

- Arrowroot Powder (2 tablespoons): Acts as a base and provides a smooth texture to the foundation.
- Shea Butter (1 tablespoon): Offers moisture and helps in achieving a creamy consistency for the foundation.
- Frankincense Essential Oil (4-5 drops): Provides skincare benefits, such as anti-inflammatory and soothing properties.
- Jojoba Oil (1 tablespoon): Balances natural oils, hydrates the skin, and aids in blending.

Tools Required:

- DOUBLE BOILER OR microwave
- Mixing bowl
- Measuring spoons
- Small container for storage

Method:

1. Homemade Version:

- MELT INGREDIENTS: Use a double boiler or microwave to melt the shea butter until it becomes liquid. Combine it with jojoba oil in a mixing bowl.
- Incorporate Arrowroot Powder: Gradually add arrowroot powder while stirring continuously to ensure an even mixture.
- Add Frankincense Essential Oil: Mix in 4-5 drops of frankincense essential oil, ensuring it is well blended for its skincare benefits.
- Test & Adjust: Apply a small amount to your skin to test the coverage and texture. Adjust arrowroot powder or essential oil quantities for desired coverage or skincare benefits.

- Storage: Transfer the foundation into a clean, small container for storage. Keep it in a cool, dry place away from direct sunlight.

Additional Tips:

- *Texture & Coverage:* Adjust arrowroot powder quantities for a matte finish or increased coverage. Increase jojoba oil for a more hydrating foundation.
- *Essential Oils:* Consider adding a drop of organic essential oil for a pleasant scent and added skincare benefits.

Caution:

- ALWAYS PERFORM A patch test on a small area of your skin before applying the foundation to ensure no adverse reactions occur.

Commercial Version:

DEVELOPING A COMMERCIAL version of this foundation might be advantageous! To modify it for commercial use:

- Additional Ingredients: Include organic cocoa butter (1 tablespoon) for enhanced skin nourishment and texture.
- Method Changes: Use professional-grade equipment for consistency in larger batches.
- Packaging Tips: Opt for eco-friendly, labeled packaging that emphasizes its organic nature. Ensure proper sealing for a longer shelf life.
- Shelf Life: The shelf life for the commercial version can be around 6-12 months if stored correctly.

Unique Selling Proposition (USP):

THIS ORGANIC FRANKINCENSE Essential Oil Foundation offers skincare benefits along with coverage, catering to those seeking both natural beauty and skincare enhancements. It promotes a radiant complexion while soothing and nourishing the skin.

Crafting cosmetics for commercial use requires compliance with safety regulations, meticulous testing, and adherence to labeling laws. Always ensure legal compliance and safety standards.

Bright Eyes: Homemade Organic Under Eye Concealer

Ingredients:

- Coconut Oil (1 tablespoon): Provides hydration and acts as a base for the concealer.
- Shea Butter (1 tablespoon): Offers moisture and helps in achieving a smooth texture for the concealer.
- Beeswax (1 tablespoon): Acts as a natural thickening agent for the concealer.
- Almond Oil (1 teaspoon): Nourishes the delicate under-eye area and aids in blending.

Tools Required:

- DOUBLE BOILER OR microwave
  - Mixing bowl
  - Measuring spoons
  - Small container for storage

Method:

1. Homemade Version:

- MELT INGREDIENTS: Use a double boiler or microwave to melt the shea butter and beeswax until they become liquid. Combine them with coconut oil in a mixing bowl.
- Incorporate Almond Oil: Gradually add almond oil while stirring continuously to ensure an even mixture and added skincare benefits.
- Blend Thoroughly: Mix the ingredients thoroughly until you achieve a smooth and consistent texture.
- Cooling and Storing: Allow the mixture to cool for a few minutes before transferring it into a small, clean container for storage.

Additional Tips:

• *Customization:* Adjust the quantities of shea butter or almond oil for a thicker or smoother consistency, according to personal preference.

• *Skin-loving Additions:* Consider adding a drop of organic vitamin E oil for added nourishment and antioxidant benefits.

Caution:

• PERFORM A PATCH test on a small area of your skin before applying the concealer to ensure no adverse reactions occur, especially since the eye area can be sensitive.

Commercial Version:

CREATING A COMMERCIAL version may be advantageous! To modify it for commercial use:

• Additional Ingredients: Include organic arrowroot powder (1 teaspoon) for enhanced coverage and a more matte finish.

• Method Changes: Use professional-grade equipment for consistency in larger batches.

• Packaging Tips: Opt for air-tight, small packaging that allows for easy application. Emphasize its organic and skin-friendly nature on the label.

• Shelf Life: The shelf life for the commercial version can be around 6-12 months if stored correctly.

Unique Selling Proposition (USP):

THIS ORGANIC UNDER Eye Concealer not only offers coverage but also contains natural ingredients that nourish and hydrate the delicate under-eye area. Its skin-loving components promote a refreshed and brightened appearance.

Crafting cosmetics for commercial use requires compliance with safety regulations, meticulous testing, and adherence to labeling laws. Always ensure legal compliance and safety standards.

Refresh & Conceal: Homemade Green Tea Infused Concealer

Ingredients:

- Coconut Oil (1 tablespoon): Serves as a base, offering hydration and aiding in blending.
- Shea Butter (1 tablespoon): Provides moisture and helps achieve a creamy texture for the concealer.
- Beeswax (1 tablespoon): Acts as a natural thickening agent for the concealer.
- Green Tea Leaves (1 teaspoon): Infuses the concoction with antioxidants and anti-inflammatory properties.

Tools Required:

- DOUBLE BOILER OR microwave
- Mixing bowl
- Fine strainer or cheesecloth
- Measuring spoons
- Small container for storage

Method:

1. Homemade Version:

- INFUSING GREEN TEA: In a double boiler or microwave, melt the shea butter and beeswax until they become liquid. Add coconut oil and green tea leaves to infuse the mixture. Let it sit for 15-20 minutes.
- Strain the Mixture: After the infusion time, strain the mixture using a fine strainer or cheesecloth to remove the green tea leaves.
- Mixing Ingredients: Return the strained mixture to heat and blend it thoroughly until well combined.
- Cooling and Storing: Allow the mixture to cool for a few minutes before transferring it into a clean, small container for storage.

Additional Tips:

• *Consistency Adjustment:* Alter the ratio of shea butter to beeswax for a thicker consistency or more beeswax for increased coverage.

• *Green Tea Concentration:* Adjust the amount of green tea leaves for a stronger infusion and increased antioxidant benefits.

Caution:

• ALWAYS PERFORM A patch test on a small area of your skin before applying the concealer to ensure no adverse reactions occur, particularly as the eye area can be sensitive.

Commercial Version:

CREATING A COMMERCIAL version of this concealer could be advantageous! To modify it for commercial use:

• Additional Ingredients: Consider adding organic arrowroot powder (1 teaspoon) for enhanced coverage and a smoother finish.

• Method Changes: Use professional-grade equipment for consistency in larger batches.

• Packaging Tips: Opt for small, airtight packaging that ensures ease of application. Highlight its organic and skin-loving properties on the label.

• Shelf Life: The shelf life for the commercial version can be around 6-12 months if stored correctly.

Unique Selling Proposition (USP):

THIS ORGANIC GREEN Tea Infused Concealer not only provides coverage but also contains antioxidant-rich green tea, offering natural skincare benefits that refresh and soothe the skin.

Crafting cosmetics for commercial use requires compliance with safety regulations, meticulous testing, and adherence to labeling laws. Always ensure legal compliance and safety standards.

Smooth Coverage: Homemade Organic Aloe Vera Concealer Stick

Ingredients:

- Aloe Vera Gel (2 tablespoons): Provides hydration and soothing properties to the skin.
- Shea Butter (1 tablespoon): Offers moisture and helps in achieving a smooth texture for the concealer stick.
- Beeswax (1 tablespoon): Acts as a natural thickening agent for the concealer stick.
- Almond Oil (1 teaspoon): Nourishes the skin and aids in blending.

Tools Required:

- DOUBLE BOILER OR microwave
  - Mixing bowl
  - Measuring spoons
  - Small container (lip balm tubes or small jars) for storage

Method:

1. Homemade Version:

- MELTING INGREDIENTS: Use a double boiler or microwave to melt the shea butter and beeswax until they become liquid. Combine them with almond oil in a mixing bowl.
- Adding Aloe Vera Gel: Gradually add aloe vera gel while stirring continuously to ensure an even mixture.
- Thorough Mixing: Blend the ingredients thoroughly until achieving a smooth and consistent texture.
- Pouring into Containers: Pour the mixture into clean, small containers like lip balm tubes or small jars for storage. Let it cool and solidify.

Additional Tips:

- *Texture Adjustment:* Alter the ratio of shea butter to beeswax for a softer or firmer texture, depending on personal preference.
- *Essential Oils:* Consider adding a drop of organic essential oil for a pleasant scent and added skincare benefits.

Caution:

- PERFORM A PATCH test on a small area of your skin before applying the concealer stick to ensure no adverse reactions occur, especially if you have sensitive skin.

Commercial Version:

CREATING A COMMERCIAL version might be beneficial! To modify it for commercial use:

- Additional Ingredients: Include organic arrowroot powder (1 teaspoon) for enhanced coverage and a more matte finish.
- Method Changes: Use professional-grade equipment for consistency in larger batches.
- Packaging Tips: Opt for convenient and hygienic packaging like twist-up tubes. Emphasize its organic nature and skin-loving properties on the label.
- Shelf Life: The shelf life for the commercial version can be around 6-12 months if stored correctly.

Unique Selling Proposition (USP):

THIS ORGANIC ALOE VERA Concealer Stick not only provides coverage but also contains soothing aloe vera gel, offering natural skincare benefits that hydrate and calm the skin.

Crafting cosmetics for commercial use requires compliance with safety regulations, meticulous testing, and adherence to labeling laws. Always ensure legal compliance and safety standards.

Rosy Glow: Homemade Organic Beetroot Blush

Ingredients:

- Beetroot Powder (2 tablespoons): Provides a natural pigment for a rosy hue.
- Arrowroot Powder (1 tablespoon): Acts as a base, helps in achieving a smooth texture.
- Kaolin Clay (1 teaspoon): Offers a matte finish and helps in blending.
- Jojoba Oil (1 teaspoon): Provides moisture and aids in the binding of ingredients.

Tools Required:

- MORTAR AND PESTLE or a coffee grinder
- Mixing bowl
- Measuring spoons
- Small container for storage

Method:

1. Homemade Version:

- GRINDING BEETROOT: Grind organic dried beetroot into a fine powder using a mortar and pestle or a coffee grinder.
- Mixing Ingredients: In a mixing bowl, combine beetroot powder, arrowroot powder, kaolin clay, and jojoba oil. Blend the ingredients thoroughly until a consistent mixture forms.
- Adjusting Consistency: If needed, add more arrowroot powder for a lighter shade or more beetroot powder for a deeper color.
- Storing the Blush: Transfer the blended mixture into a clean, small container for storage.

Additional Tips:

- *Shade Customization:* Experiment with the ratios of beetroot powder and arrowroot powder to achieve the desired blush shade.
- *Test Before Use:* Perform a patch test on a small area of your skin to ensure compatibility, especially if you have sensitive skin.

Caution:

- AVOID GETTING THE powdered mixture into your eyes. Apply the blush gently and avoid inhaling the powder.

Commercial Version:

CREATING A COMMERCIAL version could be advantageous! To modify it for commercial use:

- Additional Ingredients: Consider adding organic cocoa powder for added depth or mica for shimmer.
- Method Changes: Use professional-grade equipment for consistency in larger batches.
- Packaging Tips: Opt for compact and eco-friendly packaging that emphasizes its organic and natural attributes. Clearly state the ingredients and benefits on the packaging label.
- Shelf Life: The shelf life for the commercial version can be around 6-12 months if stored correctly.

Unique Selling Proposition (USP):

THIS ORGANIC BEETROOT Blush not only provides a natural and healthy flush of color but also contains skin-friendly ingredients that nourish and protect the skin.

Creating cosmetics for commercial use involves adherence to safety regulations, extensive testing, and compliance with labeling laws. Always ensure legal compliance and safety standards.

Floral Flush: Homemade Organic Hibiscus Petal Blush

Ingredients:

- Dried Hibiscus Petals (2 tablespoons): Provides a natural, rosy pigment.
- Arrowroot Powder (1 tablespoon): Acts as a base and helps in achieving a smooth texture.
- Kaolin Clay (1 teaspoon): Offers a matte finish and aids in blending.
- Coconut Oil (1 teaspoon): Provides moisture and helps bind the ingredients.

Tools Required:

- MORTAR AND PESTLE or a coffee grinder
- Mixing bowl
- Measuring spoons
- Small container for storage

Method:

1. Homemade Version:

- GRINDING HIBISCUS Petals: Grind organic dried hibiscus petals into a fine powder using a mortar and pestle or a coffee grinder.
- Mixing Ingredients: In a mixing bowl, combine the ground hibiscus petals, arrowroot powder, kaolin clay, and coconut oil. Mix thoroughly until a consistent mixture forms.
- Adjusting Consistency: Add more arrowroot powder for a lighter shade or more hibiscus powder for a deeper hue. Blend until the desired consistency is achieved.
- Storing the Blush: Transfer the blended mixture into a clean, small container for storage.

Additional Tips:

- *Shade Customization:* Experiment with the ratios of hibiscus petals and arrowroot powder to achieve the desired blush shade.

- *Test Before Use:* Perform a patch test on a small area of your skin to ensure compatibility, especially if you have sensitive skin.

Caution:

- AVOID GETTING THE powdered mixture into your eyes. Apply the blush gently and avoid inhaling the powder.

Commercial Version:

DEVELOPING A COMMERCIAL version might be beneficial! To adapt it for commercial use:

- Additional Ingredients: Consider adding organic beetroot powder for extra depth or mica for shimmer effects.

- Method Changes: Use professional-grade equipment for consistency in larger batches.

- Packaging Tips: Choose compact, eco-friendly packaging that highlights its organic nature. Clearly list the ingredients and benefits on the packaging label.

- Shelf Life: The shelf life for the commercial version can be around 6-12 months if stored correctly.

Unique Selling Proposition (USP):

THIS ORGANIC HIBISCUS Petal Blush provides a naturally derived blush with floral goodness that enhances your complexion while nourishing your skin.

Creating cosmetics for commercial use entails compliance with safety regulations, thorough testing, and adherence to labeling laws. Always ensure legal compliance and safety standards.

Chocolatey Glow: Homemade Organic Cocoa Powder Blush

Ingredients:

- Cocoa Powder (2 tablespoons): Provides a warm, natural tint to the blush.
- Arrowroot Powder (1 tablespoon): Acts as a base, helps achieve a smooth texture.
- Kaolin Clay (1 teaspoon): Offers a matte finish and aids in blending.
- Almond Oil (1 teaspoon): Provides moisture and helps bind the ingredients.

Tools Required:

- MORTAR AND PESTLE or a coffee grinder
- Mixing bowl
- Measuring spoons
- Small container for storage

Method:

1. Homemade Version:

GRINDING COCOA POWDER: Grind organic cocoa powder into a fine consistency using a mortar and pestle or a coffee grinder.

Mixing Ingredients: In a mixing bowl, combine the ground cocoa powder, arrowroot powder, kaolin clay, and almond oil. Thoroughly mix until a consistent blend forms.

Adjusting Consistency: If needed, add more arrowroot powder for a lighter shade or more cocoa powder for a deeper color.

Storing the Blush: Transfer the blended mixture into a clean, small container for storage.

Additional Tips:

• *Shade Customization:* Experiment with the ratios of cocoa powder and arrowroot powder to achieve the desired blush shade.

• *Patch Test:* Always perform a patch test on a small area of skin to ensure compatibility, especially for sensitive skin.

Caution:

• AVOID CONTACT WITH the eyes. Apply the blush gently and prevent inhalation of the powder.

Commercial Version:

CREATING A COMMERCIAL version might be advantageous! To adapt it for commercial use:

• Additional Ingredients: Consider adding organic beetroot powder for extra depth or mica for shimmer effects.

• Method Changes: Utilize professional-grade equipment for consistency in larger batches.

• Packaging Tips: Opt for compact, eco-friendly packaging that emphasizes its organic nature. Clearly list the ingredients and benefits on the packaging label.

• Shelf Life: The shelf life for the commercial version can be around 6-12 months if stored correctly.

Unique Selling Proposition (USP):

THIS ORGANIC COCOA Powder Blush not only provides a naturally radiant look but also contains skin-friendly ingredients that nourish and enhance your complexion.

Crafting cosmetics for commercial use involves compliance with safety regulations, thorough testing, and adherence to labeling laws. Always ensure legal compliance and safety standards.

Berry Bloom: Homemade Organic Berry Juice Blush

Ingredients:

- Mixed Organic Berry Juice (2 tablespoons): Offers natural pigmentation and a fruity hue.
- Arrowroot Powder (1 tablespoon): Acts as a base, helps achieve a smooth texture.
- Kaolin Clay (1 teaspoon): Provides a matte finish and aids in blending.
- Coconut Oil (1 teaspoon): Provides moisture and helps bind the ingredients.

Tools Required:

- MORTAR AND PESTLE or a coffee grinder
- Mixing bowl
- Measuring spoons
- Small container for storage

Method:

1. Homemade Version:

- PREPARING BERRY Juice: Extract juice from a mix of organic berries like raspberries, strawberries, or blackberries. Filter out any seeds or pulp.
- Mixing Ingredients: In a mixing bowl, combine the berry juice, arrowroot powder, kaolin clay, and coconut oil. Mix thoroughly until a consistent mixture forms.
- Adjusting Consistency: Add more arrowroot powder for a lighter shade or more berry juice for a deeper hue. Blend until the desired consistency is achieved.
- Storing the Blush: Transfer the blended mixture into a clean, small container for storage.

Additional Tips:

- *Shade Customization:* Experiment with the ratios of berry juice and arrowroot powder to achieve the desired blush shade.
- *Patch Test:* Perform a patch test on a small area of your skin to ensure compatibility, especially for sensitive skin.

Caution:

- AVOID CONTACT WITH the eyes. Apply the blush gently and prevent inhalation of the powder.

Commercial Version:

DEVELOPING A COMMERCIAL version might be beneficial! To adapt it for commercial use:

- Additional Ingredients: Consider incorporating organic beetroot powder for extra depth or mica for shimmer effects.
- Method Changes: Use professional-grade equipment for consistency in larger batches.
- Packaging Tips: Choose compact, eco-friendly packaging that highlights its organic nature. Clearly list the ingredients and benefits on the packaging label.
- Shelf Life: The shelf life for the commercial version can be around 6-12 months if stored correctly.

Unique Selling Proposition (USP):

THIS ORGANIC BERRY Juice Blush not only provides a vibrant blush but also harnesses the natural goodness of berries, offering a fresh and nourishing alternative for a radiant look.

Crafting cosmetics for commercial use involves compliance with safety regulations, thorough testing, and adherence to labeling laws. Always ensure legal compliance and safety standards.

Rosy Radiance: Organic Rosewater Blush

Ingredients:

- Organic Rosewater (3 tablespoons): Provides a gentle, refreshing base and imparts a delicate floral aroma.
- Arrowroot Powder (1 tablespoon): Serves as a base for texture and helps in achieving the desired consistency.
- Hibiscus Powder (1 teaspoon): Offers natural pigment and a lovely blush tone.
- Jojoba Oil (1 teaspoon): Adds moisturizing properties and helps in blending.

Tools Required:

- MIXING BOWL
  - Measuring spoons
  - Whisk or spoon for stirring
  - Small container for storage

Method:

1. Homemade Version:

COMBINING INGREDIENTS: In a mixing bowl, pour the organic rosewater.

Adding Powders: Gradually add the arrowroot powder and hibiscus powder into the rosewater while stirring continuously to avoid clumps.

Incorporating Jojoba Oil: Pour in the jojoba oil and mix until a smooth and consistent paste is formed.

Texture Adjustment: Adjust the texture by adding more arrowroot powder if a thicker consistency is desired.

Storage: Transfer the blush mixture into a clean, small container for storage.

Additional Tips:

• *Shade Control:* Adjust the blush color by varying the amount of hibiscus powder added.

• *Skin Patch Test:* Always perform a skin patch test to ensure compatibility, especially for sensitive skin.

Caution:

• APPLY THE BLUSH gently, avoiding contact with the eyes, and prevent inhalation of the powder.

Commercial Version:

CREATING A COMMERCIAL version could be advantageous. To adapt for commercial use:

• Additional Ingredients: Consider incorporating organic beetroot powder for added depth or mica for shimmer effects.

• Method Modifications: Utilize professional-grade equipment for consistency in larger batches.

• Packaging Advice: Opt for sustainable, eye-catching packaging that emphasizes its organic nature. Clearly list ingredients and benefits on the packaging label.

• Shelf Life: The commercial version, if stored properly, can have a shelf life of approximately 6-12 months.

Unique Selling Proposition (USP):

THIS ORGANIC ROSEWATER Blush harnesses the natural essence of roses, imparting a gentle, floral touch while providing a delightful blush, ensuring a radiant, organic glow.

Developing cosmetics for commercial use entails ensuring compliance with safety regulations, conducting thorough testing, and adhering to labeling laws. Always prioritize legal compliance and safety standards.

Organic Gel Magic: Homemade Gel Eyeliner

Ingredients:

- Organic Aloe Vera Gel (2 tablespoons): Provides a smooth and gel-like consistency as a base.
- Activated Charcoal Powder (1 teaspoon): Offers intense black color naturally.
- Organic Coconut Oil (1 teaspoon): Aids in moisturizing and achieving a creamy texture.
- Arrowroot Powder (1/2 teaspoon): Assists in adjusting the consistency.

Tools Required:

- MIXING BOWL
- Whisk or spoon for stirring
- Small airtight container for storage

Method:

1. Homemade Version:

- MIXING BASE: IN a mixing bowl, add organic aloe vera gel.
- Adding Color: Gradually incorporate activated charcoal powder into the gel while stirring continuously until the desired shade is achieved.
- Creamy Texture: Add organic coconut oil to the mixture and blend thoroughly to create a smooth texture.
- Texture Adjustment: If a thicker consistency is preferred, add arrowroot powder gradually and mix until well combined.
- Storage: Transfer the gel eyeliner into a clean, small airtight container for storage.

Additional Tips:

- *Consistency Control:* Adjust the thickness or creaminess by varying the amount of coconut oil or arrowroot powder used.
  - *Setting the Liner:* For a longer-lasting effect, set the gel eyeliner with a matching eyeshadow or translucent powder.

Caution:

- APPLY THE HOMEMADE gel eyeliner carefully and avoid direct contact with the eyes. If any irritation occurs, discontinue use immediately.

Commercial Version:

DEVELOPING A COMMERCIAL version can be a lucrative endeavor. To adapt for commercial use:

- Additional Ingredients: Consider adding vitamin E oil for its skin-nourishing properties or natural preservatives for longevity.
- Enhanced Packaging: Choose sleek and hygienic packaging that highlights its organic components and benefits. Ensure clear labeling of ingredients and usage instructions.
- Shelf Life: With proper storage and additional natural preservatives, the commercial version can have a shelf life of approximately 6-12 months.

Unique Selling Proposition (USP):

THIS HOMEMADE GEL EYELINER is crafted from organic ingredients, delivering a deep black hue without harmful additives, ensuring a safe and stunning eye makeup experience.

Creating cosmetics for commercial use involves adhering to safety regulations, conducting thorough testing, and meeting labeling requirements. Always prioritize safety and legal compliance.

Radiance Elixir: DIY Organic Liquid Highlighter

Ingredients:

- Organic Aloe Vera Gel (2 tablespoons): Provides a hydrating base that soothes the skin.
- Organic Jojoba Oil (1 teaspoon): Offers moisturizing properties without clogging pores.
- Mica Powder (1/4 teaspoon): Provides a shimmering effect for the highlight.
- Vitamin E Oil (1/4 teaspoon): Nourishes and supports skin health.

Tools Required:

- MIXING BOWL
- Whisk or spoon for blending
- Dropper bottle for storage

Method:

1. Homemade Version:

- BASE CREATION: IN a mixing bowl, combine organic aloe vera gel and organic jojoba oil. Mix well.
- Adding Shimmer: Gradually incorporate mica powder into the mixture, stirring continuously to evenly distribute the shimmer.
- Enhancing Skin: Add vitamin E oil to the mixture and blend thoroughly for its skin-nourishing benefits.
- Storage: Transfer the liquid highlighter into a clean dropper bottle for easy application and storage.

Additional Tips:

- *Adjust Shimmer:* Vary the amount of mica powder for a subtle or intense glow, depending on personal preference.

- *Blending with Foundation:* Mix a drop of this highlighter into your foundation for an all-over luminous look.

Caution:

- PERFORM A PATCH test before applying the liquid highlighter onto the face to ensure no adverse reactions. Discontinue use if irritation occurs.

Commercial Version:

CREATING A COMMERCIAL version involves:

- Additional Ingredients: Consider adding natural preservatives for an extended shelf life or incorporating plant-based pigments for a broader shade range.

- Packaging Considerations: Opt for a dropper bottle with a sleek design, emphasizing its organic and radiant properties. Clear labeling of ingredients and usage instructions is crucial.

- Shelf Life: With added preservatives, the commercial version can last approximately 6-12 months.

Unique Selling Proposition (USP):

THIS ORGANIC LIQUID Highlighter delivers a dazzling, natural radiance with its organic components, providing a luminous glow without harsh chemicals or additives.

When formulating cosmetics for commercial purposes, compliance with safety regulations, thorough testing, and accurate labeling are imperative.

Organic Glow Balm: Shea Butter Highlighter

Ingredients:

• ORGANIC SHEA BUTTER (2 tablespoons): Acts as a nourishing base that moisturizes and softens the skin.

• Organic Coconut Oil (1 tablespoon): Provides additional moisture and aids in blending.

• Mica Powder (1/2 teaspoon): Offers a shimmering effect for the highlight.

• Vitamin E Oil (1/2 teaspoon): Provides antioxidant properties and supports skin health.

Tools Required:

• MIXING BOWL
• Spoon for blending
• Small containers for storage

Method:

1. Homemade Version:

• MELTING THE BASE: In a mixing bowl, combine organic shea butter and organic coconut oil. Gently melt the mixture using a double boiler or microwave until fully liquefied.

• Adding Shimmer: Gradually add mica powder to the melted mixture, stirring continuously to ensure an even distribution of shimmer.

• Enhancing Skin: Incorporate vitamin E oil into the mixture, blending it thoroughly to infuse the highlighter with its skin-loving properties.

• Storage: Transfer the highlighter into clean, small containers for easy application and storage.

Additional Tips:

• *Adjust Shimmer:* Control the intensity of the highlight by varying the amount of mica powder used.

• *Blending Techniques:* Use fingertips or a makeup brush to apply and blend the highlighter onto desired areas for a natural glow.

Caution:

• PERFORM A PATCH test before applying the highlighter to the face to ensure no adverse reactions. Discontinue use if irritation occurs.

Commercial Version:

FOR A COMMERCIAL VERSION:

• Additional Ingredients: Consider incorporating natural preservatives for a longer shelf life and potentially introducing other organic oils or botanical extracts to enhance the product's appeal.

• Packaging Suggestions: Opt for sleek, compact containers or sticks for easy application. Clear labeling of ingredients and usage instructions is essential.

• Shelf Life: With added preservatives, the commercial version can typically last 6-12 months.

Unique Selling Proposition (USP):

THIS SHEA BUTTER HIGHLIGHTER offers a luxurious, organic glow enriched with natural ingredients, delivering radiance while nourishing the skin without any harsh chemicals.

Creating cosmetic products for commercial purposes involves adhering to safety regulations, product testing, and accurate labeling to ensure consumer satisfaction and safety.

Radiant Glow Elixir: Rosehip Oil Highlighter

Ingredients:

● Organic Rosehip Oil (1 tablespoon): Known for its skin-rejuvenating properties, providing hydration and a natural glow.

● Mica Powder (1/2 teaspoon): Adds shimmer and luminosity to the highlighter.

● Beeswax (1/2 teaspoon): Acts as a stabilizer for texture and consistency.

● Vitamin E Oil (1/2 teaspoon): Enhances skin health and acts as a natural preservative.

Tools Required:

● MIXING BOWL
● Spoon for blending
● Small containers for storage

Method:

1. Homemade Version:

● MELTING THE BASE: Combine organic rosehip oil and beeswax in a mixing bowl. Gently melt the mixture using a double boiler or microwave until fully liquefied.

● Adding Shimmer: Gradually incorporate mica powder into the melted mixture, stirring continuously to evenly disperse the shimmer.

● Enriching the Blend: Introduce vitamin E oil to the mixture, thoroughly blending it to enrich the highlighter with its skin-nourishing properties.

● Storage: Transfer the prepared highlighter into clean, small containers for convenient application and storage.

Additional Tips:

- *Adjusting Intensity:* Control the luminosity of the highlighter by adjusting the amount of mica powder added.

- *Application Technique:* Apply with fingertips or a makeup brush onto desired areas for a radiant, natural-looking glow.

Caution:

- CONDUCT A PATCH test before applying the highlighter to the face to ensure no adverse reactions. Cease use if any irritation occurs.

Commercial Version:

FOR A COMMERCIAL VERSION:

- Additional Ingredients: Consider adding natural preservatives to extend shelf life. Explore incorporating other organic oils or botanical extracts for added skin benefits.

- Packaging Recommendations: Opt for stylish, compact containers or sticks for effortless application. Clear labeling of ingredients and usage instructions is crucial.

- Shelf Life: With added preservatives, the commercial version may last 6-12 months.

Unique Selling Proposition (USP):

THIS ROSEHIP OIL HIGHLIGHTER presents a natural, organic solution for achieving a luminous complexion, harnessing the power of organic ingredients to provide both radiance and skincare benefits.

Developing cosmetics for commercial purposes necessitates compliance with safety standards, thorough product testing, and accurate labeling to ensure consumer safety and satisfaction.

Sun-Kissed Glow: Cocoa Powder Bronzer

Ingredients:

- Organic Cocoa Powder (2 tablespoons): Provides a warm, natural tone reminiscent of a sun-kissed look.
- Arrowroot Powder (1 tablespoon): Acts as a base and helps control oiliness on the skin.
- Ground Cinnamon (1/2 teaspoon): Adds a subtle hint of depth and warmth to the bronzer.
- Nutmeg (1/4 teaspoon): Enhances the bronzer's natural hue and adds a touch of radiance.

Tools Required:

- MIXING BOWL
- Spoon for blending
- Airtight container for storage

Method:

1. Homemade Version:

- BLENDING THE DRY Ingredients: In a mixing bowl, combine organic cocoa powder, arrowroot powder, ground cinnamon, and nutmeg. Mix thoroughly until all ingredients are evenly blended.
- Adjusting Consistency: If you desire a lighter shade, gradually add more arrowroot powder. Conversely, for a darker shade, increase the amount of cocoa powder.
- Storage: Transfer the prepared bronzer into an airtight container for storage.

Additional Tips:

• *Skin Tone Matching:* Experiment with ingredient ratios to suit various skin tones. Test the bronzer on the jawline to ensure a natural match.

• *Application Technique:* Apply lightly with a brush to areas where the sun naturally hits for a sun-kissed glow.

Caution:

• ALWAYS PERFORM A patch test before applying the bronzer to the face to check for any allergic reactions or skin sensitivity.

Commercial Version:

FOR A COMMERCIAL VERSION:

• Additional Ingredients: Consider including natural preservatives to extend shelf life. Experiment with different organic powders or oils for enhanced skincare benefits.

• Packaging Suggestions: Opt for sleek, eco-friendly packaging that's easy to use and carry. Clear labeling with ingredients, usage instructions, and skin tone suitability is crucial.

• Shelf Life: With added preservatives, the commercial version may last around 6-12 months.

Unique Selling Proposition (USP):

THE COCOA POWDER BRONZER offers an organic solution for achieving a sun-kissed complexion, harnessing the warmth of natural ingredients for a radiant and healthy-looking glow.

Creating cosmetics for commercial purposes involves adhering to safety guidelines, thorough product testing, and accurate labeling to ensure consumer satisfaction and safety.

Espresso Radiance: Coffee Grounds Bronzer

Ingredients:

- Organic Coffee Grounds (2 tablespoons): Rich in antioxidants, provides a warm and natural tanned hue.
- Arrowroot Powder (1 tablespoon): Serves as a base and helps control oiliness on the skin.
- Cocoa Powder (1/2 teaspoon): Adds depth and richness to the bronzer's shade.
- Ground Cinnamon (1/4 teaspoon): Enhances warmth and adds a subtle, natural glow.

Tools Required:

- MIXING BOWL
- Spoon for blending
- Airtight container for storage

Method:

1. Homemade Version:

- BLENDING THE DRY Ingredients: Combine organic coffee grounds, arrowroot powder, cocoa powder, and ground cinnamon in a mixing bowl. Mix until all ingredients are thoroughly blended.
- Adjusting Consistency: If you prefer a lighter shade, gradually add more arrowroot powder. For a deeper shade, increase the amount of coffee grounds.
- Storage: Transfer the prepared bronzer into an airtight container for storage.

Additional Tips:

- *Skin Tone Customization:* Experiment with ingredient ratios to match various skin tones. Always do a patch test on the jawline to ensure a natural blend.

- *Application Technique:* Gently apply the bronzer using a brush to areas where the sun naturally hits, such as the cheeks, forehead, and nose bridge.

Caution:

- PATCH TEST THE BRONZER on a small area of the skin before applying it to the face to ensure no allergic reactions or skin sensitivity.

Commercial Version:

FOR A COMMERCIAL VERSION:

- Additional Ingredients: Consider incorporating natural preservatives to prolong shelf life. Explore other organic powders or oils to add skincare benefits.

- Packaging Suggestions: Opt for eco-friendly packaging that's both functional and visually appealing. Clear labeling displaying ingredients, application guidelines, and suitability for different skin tones is essential.

- Shelf Life: With added preservatives, the commercial version can have a shelf life of approximately 6-12 months.

Unique Selling Proposition (USP):

THE COFFEE GROUNDS Bronzer presents an organic solution for achieving a sun-kissed glow, harnessing the power of natural ingredients to enhance the complexion with a warm, radiant tone.

Creating cosmetics for commercial purposes demands adherence to safety protocols, comprehensive product testing, and accurate labeling to ensure consumer satisfaction and safety.

Golden Glow: Turmeric Bronzer

Ingredients:

- Organic Turmeric Powder (1 tablespoon): Renowned for its anti-inflammatory and skin-brightening properties, offering a sun-kissed hue.
- Arrowroot Powder (1 tablespoon): Acts as a base and helps in achieving the desired consistency.
- Cinnamon Powder (1/2 teaspoon): Adds warmth and depth to the bronzer tone.
- Ground Ginger (1/4 teaspoon): Enhances the natural radiance and provides an extra glow.

Tools Required:

- MIXING BOWL
  - Spoon for blending
  - Airtight container for storage

Method:

1. Homemade Version:

- BLENDING THE DRY Ingredients: Combine organic turmeric powder, arrowroot powder, cinnamon powder, and ground ginger in a mixing bowl. Thoroughly blend the ingredients.
- Adjusting Consistency: Gradually add more arrowroot powder if you desire a lighter shade. Increase the turmeric amount for a deeper hue.
- Storage: Store the prepared bronzer in an airtight container.

Additional Tips:

• *Skin Tone Customization:* Experiment with ingredient ratios to match various skin tones. Conduct a patch test on the jawline to ensure a natural blend.

• *Application Technique:* Apply the bronzer lightly to areas where the sun naturally hits the face for a radiant and warm glow.

Caution:

• ALWAYS PERFORM A patch test on a small area of the skin before applying the bronzer to the face to avoid any allergic reactions or skin sensitivity.

Commercial Version:

FOR COMMERCIAL PRODUCTION:

• Additional Ingredients: Consider incorporating natural preservatives to extend shelf life. Explore adding organic oils or other skin-loving ingredients for enhanced skincare benefits.

• Packaging Suggestions: Opt for sustainable packaging that communicates product benefits clearly. Transparent labeling displaying ingredients, application guidelines, and suitability for various skin tones is essential.

• Shelf Life: With added preservatives, the commercial version can have a shelf life of approximately 6-12 months.

Unique Selling Proposition (USP):

THE TURMERIC BRONZER presents an organic, skin-friendly solution for achieving a warm, sun-kissed glow while leveraging the natural goodness of turmeric renowned for its skin-brightening properties.

Developing cosmetics for commercial purposes necessitates adhering to safety regulations, conducting comprehensive product testing, and ensuring accurate labeling for consumer satisfaction and safety.

Dewy Freshness: Aloe Vera Setting Spray

Ingredients:

- Organic Aloe Vera Juice (2 tablespoons): Provides hydration and acts as a base for the spray.
- Organic Rose Water (2 tablespoons): Offers a refreshing scent and assists in setting makeup.
- Organic Vegetable Glycerin (1/2 teaspoon): Enhances moisture retention, providing a dewy finish.
- Witch Hazel (1/2 teaspoon): Acts as a natural astringent to tighten pores and lock makeup in place.

Tools Required:

- SPRAY BOTTLE
- Funnel (for easy pouring)
- Mixing bowl

Method:

1. Homemade Version:

- PREPARATION: IN a mixing bowl, combine organic aloe vera juice and rose water.
- Add Witch Hazel: Slowly pour witch hazel into the mixture while stirring gently.
- Incorporate Glycerin: Add organic vegetable glycerin and mix well until all ingredients are thoroughly combined.
- Pour into Spray Bottle: Use a funnel to pour the solution into a clean spray bottle.
- Shake Well: Shake the bottle before each use to ensure the ingredients are properly mixed.

• Application: Spritz the setting spray onto the face after applying makeup. Hold the bottle approximately 6-8 inches away from the face while spraying.

Additional Tips:

• *Customization:* Adjust the ratios slightly to suit your skin type or preference for a more dewy or matte finish.

• *Storage:* Store the setting spray in a cool, dry place away from direct sunlight to prolong its shelf life.

Caution:

• WHILE THESE INGREDIENTS are generally safe, perform a patch test on a small area of the skin to check for any adverse reactions before applying it to the face extensively.

Commercial Version:

FOR COMMERCIAL PRODUCTION:

• Shelf Life: With the addition of natural preservatives, the commercial version can have a shelf life of around 6-12 months.

• Packaging Tips: Choose a spray bottle with a fine mist nozzle for an even application. Labeling should include usage instructions and a list of ingredients for consumer awareness.

• Ingredients Addition: Consider incorporating natural preservatives for a longer shelf life in commercial production.

Unique Selling Proposition (USP):

THIS ALOE VERA SETTING Spray combines organic ingredients to set makeup while providing a refreshing and hydrating experience, distinguishing itself as a natural and skin-friendly option in the setting spray market.

Refreshing Green Tea Glow: DIY Setting Spray

Ingredients:

- Organic Green Tea (1 bag or 1 teaspoon loose tea): Rich in antioxidants, it helps soothe and revitalize the skin.
- Organic Aloe Vera Gel (2 tablespoons): Provides hydration and helps set the makeup.
- Organic Vegetable Glycerin (1/2 teaspoon): Locks in moisture, leaving a dewy finish.
- Distilled Water (1/2 cup): Acts as the base of the spray.

Tools Required:

- Small saucepan
- Spray bottle
- Fine mesh strainer
- Funnel (for easy pouring)
- Mixing bowl

Method:

1. Homemade Version:

- PREPARE GREEN TEA: Heat distilled water in a saucepan until it just begins to simmer. Remove from heat, add the green tea bag or loose tea, and steep for 5-10 minutes. Allow it to cool to room temperature.
- Mix Ingredients: In a mixing bowl, combine the organic aloe vera gel and vegetable glycerin.
- Strain Green Tea: Once cooled, strain the green tea into the mixing bowl with the aloe vera gel and glycerin mixture. Mix well.
- Pour into Spray Bottle: Use a funnel to pour the solution into a clean spray bottle.

• Shake Well: Shake the bottle before each use to ensure the ingredients are well blended.

• Application: Close eyes and lightly spritz the setting spray onto the face after applying makeup. Hold the bottle about 6-8 inches away from the face while spraying.

Additional Tips:

• Cooling Effect: Refrigerate the setting spray for a refreshing burst when applied.

• Skin Sensitivity: Perform a patch test on a small area of the skin to ensure there are no adverse reactions before applying it to the face extensively.

Caution:

• While the ingredients are generally safe, some individuals may be sensitive to certain components. Test on a small area of skin before full application.

Commercial Version:

FOR COMMERCIAL PRODUCTION:

• Shelf Life: With the addition of natural preservatives, the commercial version can have a shelf life of around 6-12 months.

• Packaging Tips: Opt for an opaque or tinted spray bottle to protect the ingredients from light exposure. Label clearly with usage instructions and a list of organic ingredients to attract consumers seeking natural products.

• Ingredients Addition: Consider adding natural preservatives for a longer shelf life in commercial production.

Unique Selling Proposition (USP):

THIS GREEN TEA SETTING Spray harnesses the power of antioxidants and organic ingredients to set makeup while providing a refreshing and revitalizing experience, positioning itself as a natural and skin-loving alternative in the setting spray market.

Lavender Infused Glow: DIY Setting Spray

Ingredients:

- Organic Lavender Essential Oil (5-8 drops): Known for its calming properties and pleasant fragrance.
- Organic Witch Hazel (2 tablespoons): Acts as a natural astringent, aiding in setting the makeup.
- Organic Aloe Vera Gel (2 tablespoons): Provides hydration and helps set the makeup.
- Distilled Water (1/2 cup): Serves as the base of the spray.

Tools Required:

- SMALL SAUCEPAN
  - Spray bottle
  - Fine mesh strainer
  - Funnel (for easy pouring)
  - Mixing bowl

Method:

1. Homemade Version:

- PREPARE LAVENDER Solution: Heat distilled water in a saucepan until it just begins to simmer. Remove from heat, add the organic lavender essential oil, and allow it to cool to room temperature.
- Combine Ingredients: In a mixing bowl, combine the organic witch hazel and organic aloe vera gel.
- Strain Lavender Solution: Once cooled, strain the lavender-infused water into the mixing bowl with the witch hazel and aloe vera gel mixture. Mix well.
- Transfer to Spray Bottle: Use a funnel to pour the solution into a clean spray bottle.

- Shake Well: Shake the bottle before each use to ensure the ingredients are well blended.
- Application: Close eyes and lightly spritz the setting spray onto the face after applying makeup. Hold the bottle about 6-8 inches away from the face while spraying.

Additional Tips:

- *Fragrance Boost:* Add a few additional drops of lavender oil for a stronger scent if desired.
- *Cooling Sensation:* Refrigerate the setting spray for a refreshing feel upon application.

Caution:

- WHILE THE INGREDIENTS are generally safe, some individuals may be sensitive to certain components. It's advisable to test on a small area of skin before full application.

Commercial Version:

FOR COMMERCIAL PRODUCTION:
- Shelf Life: With natural preservatives, the commercial version can have a shelf life of approximately 6-12 months.
- Packaging Tips: Use an opaque or tinted spray bottle to prevent light exposure. Clearly label the bottle with usage instructions and a list of organic ingredients to appeal to customers seeking natural products.
- Ingredients Addition: Consider incorporating natural preservatives for an extended shelf life in commercial production.

Unique Selling Proposition (USP):

THIS LAVENDER INFUSED Setting Spray utilizes the calming properties of lavender oil, along with organic ingredients, to provide a soothing and refreshing setting spray that sets makeup while offering a delightful aroma, positioning itself as a natural and aromatherapeutic alternative in the setting spray market.

Natural Radiance: DIY Arrowroot Powder Face Powder

Ingredients:

● Organic Arrowroot Powder (2 tablespoons): A finely milled, lightweight powder that absorbs excess oil and provides a smooth finish.

● Organic Cornstarch (1 tablespoon): Assists in mattifying the skin and enhancing the powder's texture.

● Organic Cocoa Powder (1/2 tablespoon): Adds a subtle tint to the powder for different skin tones.

● Organic Ground Cinnamon (1/2 teaspoon): Provides a warm hue and adds a natural scent.

● Organic Ground Nutmeg (1/4 teaspoon): Offers a hint of warmth and color to the powder.

Tools Required:

● MIXING BOWL
● Spoon or whisk for mixing
● Airtight container for storage

Method:

1. Homemade Version:

● MIX DRY INGREDIENTS: In a mixing bowl, combine the organic arrowroot powder, organic cornstarch, organic cocoa powder, organic ground cinnamon, and organic ground nutmeg. Use a spoon or whisk to blend the ingredients thoroughly.

● Adjust Color (Optional): Depending on your skin tone, adjust the amount of cocoa powder or spices to achieve the desired shade. Test the color on your skin to ensure it matches.

• Transfer to Container: Once thoroughly mixed, carefully transfer the powder to an airtight container for storage. Ensure the container is clean and dry before adding the powder.

• Application: Use a makeup brush or puff to apply the powder onto the face lightly. Focus on areas that tend to get oily or need a setting powder after foundation application.

Additional Tips:

• *Customize Shades:* Experiment with the ratios of cocoa powder, cinnamon, and nutmeg to create various shades suited to different skin tones.

• *Sift Ingredients:* To achieve a smoother texture, sift the ingredients before mixing.

Caution:

• SOME INDIVIDUALS might have sensitivities to certain spices. It's advisable to do a patch test before applying the powder to the face, especially for those with sensitive skin.

Commercial Version:

FOR COMMERCIAL PRODUCTION:

• Shelf Life: When stored in a cool, dry place, this powder can have a shelf life of approximately 6-12 months.

• Packaging Tips: Use eco-friendly, refillable containers that are airtight to maintain the powder's freshness. Label the product with the ingredients used and usage instructions.

• Additional Ingredients: For commercial use, consider incorporating natural preservatives to extend shelf life and ensure product safety.

Unique Selling Proposition (USP):

THIS DIY ARROWROOT Powder Face Powder offers a natural alternative to commercial face powders, providing a customizable solution for various skin tones while utilizing organic ingredients that are gentle on the skin, making it a healthier and eco-conscious option for makeup enthusiasts.

Fresh Glow: DIY Rice Flour Face Powder

Ingredients:

- Organic Rice Flour (3 tablespoons): Rice flour acts as a gentle exfoliant and helps absorb excess oil, giving a matte finish to the skin.
- Organic Cornstarch (1 tablespoon): Provides a silky texture and aids in oil absorption, enhancing the powder's smoothness.
- Organic Arrowroot Powder (1/2 tablespoon): Enhances the powder's lightness and offers a soft, velvety feel on the skin.

Tools Required:

- MIXING BOWL
- Spoon or whisk for blending
- Clean, airtight container for storage

Method:

1. Homemade Version:

- COMBINE DRY INGREDIENTS: In a mixing bowl, blend together the organic rice flour, organic cornstarch, and organic arrowroot powder using a spoon or whisk. Ensure an even distribution of all ingredients.
- Texture Adjustment: Assess the texture of the mixture. If a finer texture is desired, blend the mixture further using a sieve to achieve a smoother consistency.
- Transfer to Container: Carefully transfer the blended powder into a clean, airtight container. Ensure the container is dry before adding the powder to prevent clumping.
- Application: Use a powder puff or makeup brush to apply the powder lightly onto the face, focusing on areas prone to oiliness or where foundation or concealer has been applied.

Additional Tips:

- *Customize Formula:* Adjust the ratio of ingredients to suit personal preferences regarding texture, coverage, or oil absorption.
  - *Scent Enhancement:* Incorporate a few drops of organic essential oils like lavender or rose for a fragrant touch (optional).

Caution:

- IT'S ADVISABLE TO perform a patch test before applying the powder to the face, especially for individuals with sensitive skin or allergies to rice-based products.

Commercial Version:

FOR COMMERCIAL PRODUCTION:

- Shelf Life: Under proper storage conditions (cool, dry place), the powder can last around 6-12 months.
- Packaging Tips: Use eco-friendly, recyclable packaging that is airtight to maintain the powder's freshness and quality. Label the container with the list of ingredients and usage instructions.
- Additional Ingredients: For commercial purposes, consider incorporating natural preservatives to extend shelf life and maintain product safety.

Unique Selling Proposition (USP):

THIS DIY RICE FLOUR Face Powder offers a natural and organic alternative to traditional face powders. It combines gentle exfoliation with oil-absorbing properties, leaving the skin with a radiant and matte finish. Its simplicity, organic components, and customizable formula make it an appealing option for those seeking a chemical-free makeup solution.

Radiant Glow: DIY Tapioca Flour Face Powder

Ingredients:

- Organic Tapioca Flour (4 tablespoons): Tapioca flour offers a silky texture, helps in oil absorption, and provides a smooth finish to the skin.
- Organic Arrowroot Powder (2 tablespoons): Enhances the softness and absorbency of the powder, contributing to a lightweight feel on the skin.

Tools Required:

- MIXING BOWL
  - Spoon or whisk for blending
  - Clean, airtight container for storage

Method:

1. Homemade Version:

- COMBINE DRY INGREDIENTS: In a mixing bowl, blend the organic tapioca flour and organic arrowroot powder thoroughly using a spoon or whisk. Ensure a uniform mixture.
  - Texture Refinement: If a finer texture is desired, sieve the blended powder to remove any lumps and achieve a smoother consistency.
  - Transfer to Container: Carefully pour the refined powder into a clean, airtight container. Make sure the container is dry to prevent moisture from affecting the powder's quality.
  - Application: Apply the powder with a brush or puff gently on the face, focusing on oily areas or over foundation for a matte finish.

Additional Tips:

- *Customization:* Adjust the quantity of ingredients to attain the preferred consistency and oil-absorbing effect.
    - *Scent Infusion:* Consider adding a few drops of organic essential oils like lavender or chamomile for a pleasing fragrance (optional).

Caution:

- PERFORM A PATCH test before applying the powder extensively, especially for individuals with sensitive skin or allergies to tapioca-based products.

Commercial Version:

FOR COMMERCIAL PRODUCTION:
- Shelf Life: Stored properly in a dry, cool place, the powder can retain its quality for about 6-12 months.
- Packaging Tips: Use eco-friendly, airtight containers for packaging. Label the containers with ingredient lists, usage instructions, and expiration dates.
- Additional Ingredients: For commercial purposes, consider incorporating natural preservatives to extend the product's shelf life and ensure safety.

Unique Selling Proposition (USP):

THIS DIY TAPIOCA FLOUR Face Powder offers a natural alternative to conventional face powders. Its organic components provide a smooth and oil-absorbing solution for a radiant and matte complexion. The simplicity of its formulation, along with its customizable nature, makes it an attractive option for those seeking organic skincare products.

DIY Organic Pressed Eyeshadow Palette Recipe

Ingredients

Base Ingredients

- Arrowroot Powder: Adds a smooth texture to the eyeshadow. It helps with oil absorption and creates a matte finish. (*Quantity: 2 tablespoons*)
- Kaolin Clay: This clay helps with adhesion and gives the eyeshadow its fine texture. It also absorbs excess oil. (*Quantity: 1 tablespoon*)
- Jojoba Oil: A moisturizing oil that helps bind the ingredients together, providing a creamy consistency. (*Quantity: 1 teaspoon*)

Pigments

- MICA POWDERS (VARIOUS Colors): Provides the color for your eyeshadows. Ensure they are cosmetic-grade and safe for use on the skin. (*Quantity: 1-2 teaspoons each color, depending on desired intensity*)

Optional Ingredients (For Scent or Extra Benefits)

- ESSENTIAL OILS: Choose skin-safe essential oils for fragrance, if desired. (*Quantity: 1-2 drops, optional*)

Tools Required

- MIXING BOWLS
  - Measuring spoons
  - Small spatula or spoon for mixing
  - Small containers or pans for pressing the eyeshadows
  - Palette case or container to store the finished eyeshadow palette

Method

Homemade Version

Step 1: Mixing the Base

IN A MIXING BOWL, COMBINE the arrowroot powder and kaolin clay.

Add jojoba oil gradually while stirring until you achieve a dough-like consistency.

Step 2: Adding Color

DIVIDE THE BASE MIXTURE into smaller portions if making multiple colors.

Add your desired mica powder to each portion. Mix well until the color is evenly distributed.

Step 3: Pressing the Eyeshadows

PLACE THE COLORED MIXTURE into small containers or pans, pressing it firmly to shape.

Allow the eyeshadows to dry and set for at least 24 hours.

Additional Tips

● EXPERIMENT WITH different color combinations by mixing various mica powders.

● Use a pressing tool or coin wrapped in a cloth to firmly press the eyeshadows for a smoother finish.

Caution

● AVOID USING NON-cosmetic grade pigments or unsafe ingredients on the skin.

Commercial Version

FOR COMMERCIAL PRODUCTION, the process remains the same, but you may need to consider:

- Ingredients for Commercial Version:

- Titanium Dioxide: To enhance color opacity and brightness. *(Quantity: 1/2 teaspoon)*

- Preservatives: For extending shelf life. Opt for natural preservatives suitable for cosmetics. *(Quantity: As per manufacturer's recommendation)*

Adjustments for Commercial Version

- ENSURE ALL INGREDIENTS meet cosmetic regulations and safety standards.
- Properly label ingredients, including preservatives and additives, for consumer awareness and safety.

Shelf Life

- HOMEMADE: APPROXIMATELY 6-12 months if stored in a cool, dry place.
- Commercial: Varies based on preservatives used and packaging. Typically 1-2 years.

Packaging Tips for Commercial Use

- USE AIRTIGHT, STERILE, and easily sealable packaging.
- Consider eco-friendly and attractive packaging to appeal to consumers.

Unique Selling Proposition (USP)

- EMPHASIZE ORGANIC, natural ingredients and cruelty-free production.
  - Highlight the customizable nature of the palette, allowing users to create their unique shades.

Crafting an organic pressed eyeshadow palette can be a rewarding venture. Just ensure compliance with cosmetic regulations and safety standards for commercial production.

DIY Organic Loose Mineral Eyeshadow Recipe

Ingredients

Base Ingredients

- Arrowroot Powder: Known for its oil-absorbing properties, it provides a smooth texture to the eyeshadow. (*Quantity: 1 tablespoon*)
- Kaolin Clay: Helps with adhesion and gives a silky feel to the eyeshadow. It also absorbs excess oil. (*Quantity: 1 tablespoon*)
- Jojoba Oil: A natural moisturizer that binds the ingredients together, giving a creamy consistency. (*Quantity: 1 teaspoon*)

Pigments

- MICA POWDERS (VARIOUS Colors): Provides the vibrant hues for your eyeshadows. Ensure they are skin-safe and cosmetic-grade. (*Quantity: 1-2 teaspoons each color, as per desired intensity*)

Optional Ingredients (For Scent or Extra Benefits)

- ESSENTIAL OILS: Skin-safe essential oils for fragrance, if desired. (*Quantity: 1-2 drops, optional*)

Tools Required

- MIXING BOWLS
  - Measuring spoons
  - Small spatula or spoon for mixing
  - Airtight containers or jars for storage

Method

Homemade Version

Step 1: Mixing the Base

IN A MIXING BOWL, COMBINE arrowroot powder and kaolin clay.

Gradually add jojoba oil while stirring until you achieve a soft, dough-like consistency.

Step 2: Adding Color

DIVIDE THE BASE MIXTURE into smaller portions if making multiple colors.

Incorporate the desired mica powder into each portion. Mix thoroughly until the color is evenly distributed.

Step 3: Storing the Eyeshadow

STORE YOUR LOOSE MINERAL eyeshadow in a clean, airtight container or jar.

Additional Tips

● EXPERIMENT WITH different color combinations by mixing various mica powders to create your unique shades.

● Use a small, clean makeup brush to apply the loose mineral eyeshadow for precise application.

Caution

● ENSURE ALL INGREDIENTS used are skin-safe and free from harmful additives or contaminants.

Commercial Version

FOR COMMERCIAL PRODUCTION, the process remains similar, but consider:

Adjustments for Commercial Version

- INGREDIENTS FOR Commercial Version:

  - Titanium Dioxide: Enhances color opacity and brightness. *(Quantity: 1/2 teaspoon)*

  - Magnesium Stearate: Improves texture and adhesion of the eyeshadow. *(Quantity: 1/4 teaspoon)*

Shelf Life

- HOMEMADE: APPROXIMATELY 6-12 months if stored in a cool, dry place.
  - Commercial: Varies based on preservatives used and packaging. Typically 1-2 years.

Packaging Tips for Commercial Use

- OPT FOR ECO-FRIENDLY, airtight, and attractive packaging that reflects the organic nature of the product.
  - Clearly label all ingredients and their proportions for customer awareness.

Unique Selling Proposition (USP)

- HIGHLIGHT THE ORGANIC, natural ingredients and the customizable nature of the loose mineral eyeshadow.
  - Emphasize the cruelty-free production process and the versatility of the product for creating various eye looks.

Creating your organic loose mineral eyeshadow is a wonderful way to craft personalized shades while ensuring the use of natural ingredients. For commercial production, ensure compliance with cosmetic regulations and safety standards while accentuating the product's organic qualities and versatility.

DIY Organic Cocoa Powder Eyeshadow Recipe

Ingredients

Base Ingredients

- Arrowroot Powder: Known for its oil-absorbing properties, providing a smooth texture to the eyeshadow. *(Quantity: 1 tablespoon)*
- Kaolin Clay: Helps with adhesion and gives a velvety feel to the eyeshadow. It also absorbs excess oil. *(Quantity: 1 tablespoon)*
- Jojoba Oil: Acts as a natural binder, giving a creamy consistency to the eyeshadow. *(Quantity: 1 teaspoon)*
- Cocoa Powder: Provides a natural brown hue and a subtle fragrance. *(Quantity: 1-2 teaspoons, depending on desired shade intensity)*

Optional Ingredients (For Scent or Extra Benefits)

- ESSENTIAL OILS: Skin-safe essential oils for fragrance, if desired. *(Quantity: 1-2 drops, optional)*

Tools Required

- MIXING BOWLS
  - Measuring spoons
  - Small spatula or spoon for mixing
  - Airtight containers or jars for storage

Method

Homemade Version

Step 1: Mixing the Base

IN A MIXING BOWL, COMBINE arrowroot powder and kaolin clay.

Gradually add jojoba oil while stirring until achieving a soft, dough-like consistency.

Step 2: Adding Color and Fragrance

DIVIDE THE BASE MIXTURE into smaller portions if creating multiple shades.

Incorporate cocoa powder into each portion for the desired brown hue.

Optionally, add a drop or two of skin-safe essential oils for fragrance. Mix thoroughly until the color and scent are evenly distributed.

Step 3: Storing the Eyeshadow

STORE THE COCOA POWDER eyeshadow in a clean, airtight container or jar.

Additional Tips

• EXPERIMENT WITH cocoa powder quantities to adjust the eyeshadow's darkness or lightness.

• Conduct a patch test to ensure the cocoa powder doesn't cause any irritation before applying it to the eyes.

Caution

• AVOID CONTACT WITH eyes and discontinue use if any irritation occurs.

• Ensure all ingredients are organic and free from additives or contaminants.

Commercial Version

FOR COMMERCIAL PRODUCTION, consider:

Adjustments for Commercial Version

- INGREDIENTS FOR Commercial Version:

  - Titanium Dioxide: Enhances color opacity and brightness. *(Quantity: 1/2 teaspoon)*

  - Magnesium Stearate: Improves texture and adhesion of the eyeshadow. *(Quantity: 1/4 teaspoon)*

Shelf Life

- HOMEMADE: APPROXIMATELY 6-12 months if stored in a cool, dry place.
  - Commercial: Varies based on preservatives used and packaging. Typically 1-2 years.

Packaging Tips for Commercial Use

- OPT FOR ECO-FRIENDLY, airtight, and visually appealing packaging to attract customers.
  - Clearly label ingredients and usage instructions for consumer awareness and safety.

Unique Selling Proposition (USP)

- EMPHASIZE THE ORGANIC and natural qualities of the cocoa powder eyeshadow.
  - Highlight the versatility of the shade, suitable for various eye looks, and the subtle fragrance imparted by cocoa powder.

Creating an organic cocoa powder eyeshadow offers a natural alternative for eye makeup enthusiasts. For commercial production, adhere to cosmetic regulations, emphasizing the product's organic nature and versatility while ensuring safety and quality standards.

DIY Organic Turmeric Eyeshadow Recipe

Ingredients

Base Ingredients

- Arrowroot Powder: Renowned for its oil-absorbing properties, providing a smooth texture to the eyeshadow. *(Quantity: 1 tablespoon)*
- Kaolin Clay: Enhances adhesion and imparts a silky feel to the eyeshadow. It also helps in absorbing excess oil. *(Quantity: 1 tablespoon)*
- Jojoba Oil: Acts as a natural binder, contributing to a creamy consistency in the eyeshadow. *(Quantity: 1 teaspoon)*
- Turmeric Powder: Offers a beautiful yellow pigment and contains antioxidants known for skin benefits. *(Quantity: 1-2 teaspoons, depending on desired shade intensity)*

Optional Ingredients (For Scent or Extra Benefits)

- ESSENTIAL OILS: Skin-safe essential oils for fragrance, if desired. *(Quantity: 1-2 drops, optional)*

Tools Required

- MIXING BOWLS
  - Measuring spoons
  - Small spatula or spoon for mixing
  - Airtight containers or jars for storage

Method

Homemade Version

Step 1: Mixing the Base

IN A MIXING BOWL, COMBINE arrowroot powder and kaolin clay.

Gradually add jojoba oil while stirring until achieving a soft, dough-like consistency.

Step 2: Adding Color and Fragrance

DIVIDE THE BASE MIXTURE into smaller portions if creating multiple shades.

Mix in turmeric powder into each portion to achieve the desired yellow hue.

Optionally, add a drop or two of skin-safe essential oils for a pleasant fragrance. Mix well until the color and scent are evenly distributed.

Step 3: Storing the Eyeshadow

STORE THE TURMERIC eyeshadow in a clean, airtight container or jar.

Additional Tips

• ADJUST THE QUANTITY of turmeric powder for different shades of yellow.

• Perform a patch test to ensure the turmeric doesn't cause any skin irritation before applying it near the eyes.

Caution

• AVOID CONTACT WITH eyes and discontinue use if any irritation occurs.

• Ensure the turmeric used is organic to maintain the purity of the eyeshadow.

Commercial Version

FOR COMMERCIAL PRODUCTION, consider:

Adjustments for Commercial Version

- INGREDIENTS FOR Commercial Version:

  - Titanium Dioxide: Enhances color opacity and brightness. *(Quantity: 1/2 teaspoon)*

  - Magnesium Stearate: Improves texture and adhesion of the eyeshadow. *(Quantity: 1/4 teaspoon)*

Shelf Life

- HOMEMADE: APPROXIMATELY 6-12 months if stored in a cool, dry place.
  - Commercial: Varies based on preservatives used and packaging. Typically 1-2 years.

Packaging Tips for Commercial Use

- OPT FOR VISUALLY appealing, airtight, and eco-friendly packaging to attract customers.
  - Clearly label ingredients and usage instructions for consumer awareness and safety.

Unique Selling Proposition (USP)

- HIGHLIGHT THE ORGANIC and natural nature of the turmeric eyeshadow.
  - Emphasize the antioxidant benefits of turmeric for the skin, offering both color and skincare benefits in one product.

Creating an organic turmeric eyeshadow allows for a natural and vibrant yellow eye makeup option. For commercial production, follow cosmetic regulations while highlighting the product's organic quality and skincare benefits. Ensure safety and quality standards for a successful and appealing commercial product.

DIY Organic Brown Sugar Lip Scrub

Ingredients

- Organic Brown Sugar: Acts as a natural exfoliant, removing dead skin cells from lips. *(Quantity: 2 tablespoons)*
- Organic Coconut Oil: Provides hydration and nourishment to the lips. *(Quantity: 1 tablespoon)*
- Organic Honey: Offers antibacterial properties and further moisturizes the lips. *(Quantity: 1 teaspoon)*
- Organic Vanilla Extract or Essential Oil: Adds a pleasant scent. *(Quantity: 1-2 drops, optional)*

Tools Required

- MIXING BOWL
  - Measuring spoons
  - Small jar or container for storage

Method

Homemade Version

Step 1: Mixing the Ingredients

IN A MIXING BOWL, COMBINE the brown sugar, coconut oil, and honey.

Add the vanilla extract or essential oil if desired for fragrance.

Mix all the ingredients thoroughly until well combined.

Step 2: Storing the Lip Scrub

TRANSFER THE PREPARED lip scrub into a clean, airtight jar or container for storage.

Additional Tips

● BEFORE APPLYING the scrub, wet your lips slightly to make the exfoliation gentler.

  ● Use the lip scrub once or twice a week for smoother, softer lips.

Caution

● AVOID USING THE lip scrub if you have any allergies to the ingredients.

  ● Don't use the scrub on cracked or injured lips.

Commercial Version

FOR COMMERCIAL PRODUCTION, consider:

Adjustments for Commercial Version

● INGREDIENTS FOR Commercial Version:

  ● Vitamin E Oil: Acts as a natural preservative and adds extra nourishment to the lips. *(Quantity: 1 teaspoon)*

  ● Beeswax: Helps in solidifying the lip scrub and provides a smoother texture. *(Quantity: 1 teaspoon)*

Shelf Life

● HOMEMADE: APPROXIMATELY 2-3 months if stored in a cool, dry place.

  ● Commercial: Varies based on preservatives used and packaging. Typically 6-12 months.

Packaging Tips for Commercial Use

- OPT FOR HYGIENIC and appealing packaging in small jars or tubes.
  - Include clear and concise instructions on usage and storage.

Unique Selling Proposition (USP)

- HIGHLIGHT THE USE of organic ingredients for natural and safe lip care.
  - Emphasize the dual action of exfoliation and hydration for soft, smooth lips.

Creating an organic brown sugar lip scrub offers a natural way to exfoliate and moisturize lips. For commercial production, follow cosmetic regulations, emphasize organic qualities, and ensure product safety and quality for a successful and appealing commercial product.

DIY Organic Honey Lip Scrub

Ingredients

- Organic Brown Sugar: Acts as a gentle exfoliant, removing dead skin cells. (*Quantity: 2 tablespoons*)
- Organic Coconut Oil: Provides moisture and nourishment to the lips. (*Quantity: 1 tablespoon*)
- Organic Honey: Offers antibacterial properties and further moisturizes the lips. (*Quantity: 1 tablespoon*)
- Organic Vanilla Extract or Essential Oil: Adds a pleasant scent. (*Quantity: 1-2 drops, optional*)

Tools Required

- MIXING BOWL
- Measuring spoons
- Small jar or container for storage

Method

Homemade Version

Step 1: Mixing the Ingredients

IN A MIXING BOWL, COMBINE the brown sugar, coconut oil, and honey.

Add the vanilla extract or essential oil if desired for fragrance.

Mix all the ingredients thoroughly until well combined.

Step 2: Storing the Lip Scrub

TRANSFER THE PREPARED lip scrub into a clean, airtight jar or container for storage.

Additional Tips

● BEFORE APPLYING the scrub, dampen your lips slightly to make the exfoliation gentler.

● Use the lip scrub once or twice a week for softer, smoother lips.

Caution

● IF YOU HAVE ANY allergies to the ingredients, avoid using the lip scrub.

● Don't use the scrub on cracked or injured lips.

Commercial Version

FOR COMMERCIAL PRODUCTION, consider:

Adjustments for Commercial Version

● INGREDIENTS FOR Commercial Version:

● Vitamin E Oil: Acts as a natural preservative and provides extra nourishment to the lips. *(Quantity: 1 teaspoon)*

● Beeswax: Helps solidify the lip scrub and provides a smoother texture. *(Quantity: 1 teaspoon)*

Shelf Life

● HOMEMADE: APPROXIMATELY 2-3 months if stored in a cool, dry place.

● Commercial: Varies based on preservatives used and packaging. Typically 6-12 months.

Packaging Tips for Commercial Use

● OPT FOR HYGIENIC and appealing packaging in small jars or tubes.

● Clearly state usage instructions and storage recommendations on the packaging.

Unique Selling Proposition (USP)

● EMPHASIZE THE USE of organic ingredients for natural and safe lip care.

● Highlight the dual action of exfoliation and hydration for softer, smoother lips.

Creating an organic honey lip scrub offers a natural way to exfoliate and moisturize lips. For commercial production, follow cosmetic regulations, highlight organic qualities, ensure product safety and quality for an appealing commercial product.

DIY Organic Coffee Grounds Lip Scrub

Ingredients

- Organic Coffee Grounds: Acts as a natural exfoliant, removing dead skin cells. *(Quantity: 1 tablespoon)*
- Organic Coconut Oil: Provides moisture and nourishment to the lips. *(Quantity: 1 tablespoon)*
- Organic Brown Sugar: Offers gentle exfoliation and helps in removing dry skin. *(Quantity: 1 tablespoon)*
- Organic Honey: Provides antibacterial properties and further moisturizes the lips. *(Quantity: 1 teaspoon)*

Tools Required

- MIXING BOWL
- Measuring spoons
- Small jar or container for storage

Method

Homemade Version

Step 1: Mixing the Ingredients

IN A MIXING BOWL, COMBINE the coffee grounds, coconut oil, brown sugar, and honey.

Mix all the ingredients thoroughly until well combined.

Step 2: Storing the Lip Scrub

TRANSFER THE PREPARED lip scrub into a clean, airtight jar or container for storage.

Additional Tips

● GENTLY MASSAGE THE lip scrub onto damp lips in circular motions for effective exfoliation.

● Rinse off the scrub with warm water and follow up with a lip balm for extra hydration.

Caution

● AVOID USING THE lip scrub on cracked or injured lips.

● If you're allergic to any of the ingredients, refrain from using the scrub.

Commercial Version

FOR COMMERCIAL PRODUCTION, consider:

Adjustments for Commercial Version

● INGREDIENTS FOR Commercial Version:

● Vitamin E Oil: Acts as a natural preservative and provides extra nourishment to the lips. *(Quantity: 1 teaspoon)*

● Beeswax: Helps solidify the lip scrub and provides a smoother texture. *(Quantity: 1 teaspoon)*

Shelf Life

● HOMEMADE: APPROXIMATELY 2-3 months if stored in a cool, dry place.

● Commercial: Varies based on preservatives used and packaging. Typically 6-12 months.

Packaging Tips for Commercial Use

● OPT FOR HYGIENIC and visually appealing packaging in small jars or tubes.

● Clearly state usage instructions and storage recommendations on the packaging.

Unique Selling Proposition (USP)

● HIGHLIGHT THE USE of organic ingredients for natural and safe lip care.

● Emphasize the dual action of exfoliation with coffee grounds and moisture with coconut oil for smoother lips.

Creating an organic coffee grounds lip scrub offers a natural way to exfoliate and moisturize lips. For commercial production, follow cosmetic regulations, emphasize organic qualities, ensure product safety, and quality for an appealing commercial product.

DIY Organic Cornstarch Setting Powder

Ingredients

- Organic Cornstarch: Acts as a base for the setting powder, absorbing excess oil and providing a matte finish. *(Quantity: 2 tablespoons)*
- Organic Arrowroot Powder: Enhances the smoothness and absorption of the powder. *(Quantity: 1 tablespoon)*
- Organic Cocoa Powder or Cinnamon Powder (for darker skin tones): Adds a tint to match various skin tones. *(Quantity: 1/2 - 1 teaspoon, optional)*

Tools Required

- MIXING BOWL
  - Measuring spoons
  - Small container for storage

Method

Homemade Version

Step 1: Mixing the Ingredients

IN A MIXING BOWL, COMBINE the cornstarch and arrowroot powder. Optionally, if you desire a tinted setting powder, add cocoa powder or cinnamon powder and mix well to blend evenly.

Step 2: Storing the Setting Powder

TRANSFER THE PREPARED setting powder into a clean, airtight container for storage.

Additional Tips

- USE A SMALL MAKEUP brush to apply the setting powder lightly over foundation or directly onto clean skin for a matte finish.
  - Adjust the quantity of cocoa powder or cinnamon powder to match your skin tone.

Caution

- AVOID INHALATION of the powder during application.
  - Discontinue use if any irritation occurs.

Commercial Version

FOR COMMERCIAL PRODUCTION, consider:

Adjustments for Commercial Version

- INGREDIENTS FOR Commercial Version:

  - Kaolin Clay: Enhances oil absorption and improves the texture of the setting powder. *(Quantity: 1 tablespoon)*

  - Titanium Dioxide: Provides opacity and brightness to the powder. *(Quantity: 1/2 teaspoon)*

Shelf Life

- HOMEMADE: APPROXIMATELY 6-12 months if stored in a cool, dry place.
  - Commercial: Varies based on preservatives used and packaging. Typically 1-2 years.

Packaging Tips for Commercial Use

● USE HYGIENIC, AIRTIGHT, and visually appealing packaging in containers suitable for easy application.

● Clearly label ingredients, usage instructions, and skin tone suitability on the packaging.

Unique Selling Proposition (USP)

● EMPHASIZE THE USE of organic ingredients for a natural and skin-friendly setting powder.

● Highlight the customizable nature of the powder with tint options for various skin tones.

Creating an organic cornstarch setting powder offers a natural way to set makeup and control shine. For commercial production, ensure compliance with cosmetic regulations, emphasize organic qualities, and focus on product safety and quality for an appealing commercial product.

DIY Organic Rice Powder Setting Powder

Ingredients

- Organic Rice Flour: Acts as the base for the setting powder, providing a smooth finish and oil absorption. *(Quantity: 2 tablespoons)*
  - Organic Arrowroot Powder: Enhances the texture and helps in oil absorption. *(Quantity: 1 tablespoon)*
  - Organic Cornstarch: Further aids in oil absorption and mattifies the skin. *(Quantity: 1 tablespoon)*
  - Organic Cocoa Powder or Cinnamon Powder (for darker skin tones): Adds a tint to match various skin tones. *(Quantity: 1/2 - 1 teaspoon, optional)*

Tools Required

- MIXING BOWL
  - Measuring spoons
  - Small container for storage

Method

Homemade Version

Step 1: Mixing the Ingredients

IN A MIXING BOWL, COMBINE the rice flour, arrowroot powder, and cornstarch.

Optionally, if desired, add cocoa powder or cinnamon powder for tint and mix well to ensure an even distribution.

Step 2: Storing the Setting Powder

TRANSFER THE PREPARED setting powder into a clean, airtight container for storage.

Additional Tips

• APPLY THE SETTING powder lightly with a makeup brush over foundation or directly onto clean skin to set makeup and control shine.

• Adjust the quantity of cocoa powder or cinnamon powder based on your skin tone for a perfect match.

Caution

• AVOID INHALATION of the powder during application.

• Discontinue use if any irritation occurs.

Commercial Version

FOR COMMERCIAL PRODUCTION, consider:

Adjustments for Commercial Version

• INGREDIENTS FOR Commercial Version:

• Kaolin Clay: Enhances oil absorption and improves the texture of the setting powder. *(Quantity: 1 tablespoon)*

• Titanium Dioxide: Provides opacity and brightness to the powder. *(Quantity: 1/2 teaspoon)*

Shelf Life

• HOMEMADE: APPROXIMATELY 6-12 months if stored in a cool, dry place.

• Commercial: Varies based on preservatives used and packaging. Typically 1-2 years.

Packaging Tips for Commercial Use

- USE HYGIENIC, AIRTIGHT, and visually appealing packaging in containers suitable for easy application.
  - Clearly label ingredients, usage instructions, and skin tone suitability on the packaging.

Unique Selling Proposition (USP)

- EMPHASIZE THE USE of organic ingredients for a natural and skin-friendly setting powder.
  - Highlight the customizable nature of the powder with tint options for various skin tones.

Crafting an organic rice powder setting powder offers a natural way to set makeup and control shine. For commercial production, ensure compliance with cosmetic regulations, emphasize organic qualities, and focus on product safety and quality for an appealing commercial product.

DIY Organic Tapioca Flour Setting Powder

Ingredients

- Organic Tapioca Flour: Serves as the base for the setting powder, providing a smooth and silky finish to the skin. *(Quantity: 2 tablespoons)*
- Organic Arrowroot Powder: Enhances texture and helps in oil absorption, preventing a shiny complexion. *(Quantity: 1 tablespoon)*
- Organic Cornstarch: Assists in oil absorption and mattifies the skin, contributing to a flawless finish. *(Quantity: 1 tablespoon)*
- Organic Cocoa Powder or Cinnamon Powder (for darker skin tones): Provides a tint to match various skin tones. *(Quantity: 1/2 - 1 teaspoon, optional)*

Tools Required

- MIXING BOWL
  - Measuring spoons
  - Small container for storage

Method

Homemade Version

Step 1: Mixing the Ingredients

IN A MIXING BOWL, COMBINE tapioca flour, arrowroot powder, and cornstarch.

Optionally, for a tinted powder, add cocoa powder or cinnamon powder and mix thoroughly for an even distribution.

Step 2: Storing the Setting Powder

TRANSFER THE PREPARED setting powder into a clean, airtight container for storage.

Additional Tips

• GENTLY APPLY THE setting powder using a makeup brush over foundation or directly onto clean skin to set makeup and control shine.
  • Adjust the quantity of cocoa powder or cinnamon powder to match your skin tone for a seamless finish.

Caution

• AVOID INHALING THE powder during application.
  • Discontinue use if any skin irritation occurs.

Commercial Version

FOR COMMERCIAL PRODUCTION, consider:

Adjustments for Commercial Version

• INGREDIENTS FOR Commercial Version:

  • Kaolin Clay: Improves oil absorption and refines texture. *(Quantity: 1 tablespoon)*

  • Titanium Dioxide: Adds opacity and brightness to the powder. *(Quantity: 1/2 teaspoon)*

Shelf Life

• HOMEMADE: APPROXIMATELY 6-12 months if stored in a cool, dry place.

● Commercial: Varies based on preservatives used and packaging. Typically 1-2 years.

Packaging Tips for Commercial Use

● USE HYGIENIC, AIRTIGHT, and visually appealing packaging in containers suitable for easy application.

● Clearly label ingredients, usage instructions, and skin tone suitability on the packaging.

Unique Selling Proposition (USP)

● EMPHASIZE THE USE of organic ingredients for a natural and skin-friendly setting powder.

● Highlight the customizable nature of the powder with tint options for various skin tones.

Crafting an organic tapioca flour setting powder provides a natural way to set makeup and achieve a matte finish. For commercial production, ensure compliance with cosmetic regulations, emphasize organic qualities, and focus on product safety and quality for an appealing commercial product.

DIY Organic Micellar Water: Gentle Cleansing for Radiant Skin

Ingredients

- Organic Witch Hazel: Acts as an astringent to cleanse and tone the skin. (*Quantity: 1/2 cup*)
- Organic Rose Water: Offers hydration and a soothing effect on the skin. (*Quantity: 1/4 cup*)
- Organic Glycerin: Provides moisture and helps maintain skin hydration. (*Quantity: 1 tablespoon*)
- Organic Jojoba Oil or Sweet Almond Oil: Offers nourishment and balances skin oils. (*Quantity: 1 teaspoon*)
- Distilled Water: Serves as a base and diluting agent. (*Quantity: 1 cup*)

Tools Required

- MIXING BOWL
- Measuring cups and spoons
- Clean, airtight container for storage
- Funnel (optional)

Method

Homemade Version

Step 1: Mixing the Ingredients

IN A MIXING BOWL, COMBINE witch hazel, rose water, glycerin, and jojoba oil (or sweet almond oil).

Slowly add distilled water to the mixture, stirring continuously to ensure thorough mixing.

Step 2: Storing the Micellar Water

CAREFULLY POUR THE prepared micellar water into a clean, airtight container. Use a funnel for ease, if needed.

Seal the container tightly.

Additional Tips

● TO USE, SATURATE a cotton pad with micellar water and gently swipe it across your face to remove makeup and impurities.

● Shake the bottle before each use to ensure the ingredients are well blended.

Caution

● AVOID CONTACT WITH eyes. If irritation occurs, rinse thoroughly with water.

Commercial Version

FOR COMMERCIAL PRODUCTION, consider:

Adjustments for Commercial Version

● INGREDIENTS FOR Commercial Version:

● Preservatives: Opt for natural preservatives to prolong shelf life. *(Quantity as per manufacturer's recommendation)*

Shelf Life

● HOMEMADE: APPROXIMATELY 2-3 weeks if stored in a cool, dark place.

● Commercial: With added preservatives, shelf life can extend to 6-12 months. Ensure to comply with regulatory guidelines for shelf life claims.

Packaging Tips for Commercial Use

● USE STERILE, AIRTIGHT, and labeled bottles with dispensers for easy and hygienic use.

● Include clear instructions on usage and storage on the packaging.

Unique Selling Proposition (USP)

● HIGHLIGHT THE ORGANIC and gentle nature of the micellar water suitable for all skin types.

● Emphasize the hydrating and cleansing properties without stripping the skin of natural oils.

Creating organic micellar water at home offers a gentle and effective way to cleanse the skin. For commercial production, ensure compliance with cosmetic regulations, focus on organic qualities, and prioritize product safety and quality for a successful and appealing commercial product.

DIY Organic Aloe Vera Makeup Remover: Gentle Care for Clean Skin

Ingredients

- Organic Aloe Vera Gel: Known for its soothing and hydrating properties, it effectively removes makeup. *(Quantity: 2 tablespoons)*
- Organic Coconut Oil: Offers moisturizing benefits and aids in breaking down makeup. *(Quantity: 1 tablespoon)*
- Organic Witch Hazel: Acts as an astringent and helps cleanse the skin. *(Quantity: 1 tablespoon)*
- Distilled Water: Serves as a diluting agent. *(Quantity: 1/4 cup)*

Tools Required

- MIXING BOWL
- Measuring spoons
- Clean, airtight container for storage
- Funnel (optional)

Method

Homemade Version

Step 1: Mixing the Ingredients

IN A MIXING BOWL, COMBINE aloe vera gel, coconut oil, and witch hazel.

Slowly add distilled water to the mixture, stirring continuously to ensure thorough mixing.

Step 2: Storing the Makeup Remover

CAREFULLY POUR THE prepared makeup remover into a clean, airtight container. Use a funnel for ease, if needed.

Seal the container tightly.

Additional Tips

- SHAKE WELL BEFORE each use to ensure all ingredients are well combined.
  - Apply a small amount of the makeup remover on a cotton pad and gently wipe off makeup from the face and eyes.

Caution

- AVOID DIRECT CONTACT with eyes. Rinse thoroughly with water if contact occurs.

Commercial Version

FOR COMMERCIAL PRODUCTION, consider:

Adjustments for Commercial Version

- INGREDIENTS FOR Commercial Version:

  - Natural Preservatives: Opt for suitable natural preservatives to extend shelf life. *(Quantity as per manufacturer's recommendation)*

Shelf Life

- HOMEMADE: APPROXIMATELY 2-3 weeks if stored in a cool, dark place.

• Commercial: With added natural preservatives, shelf life can extend to 6-12 months. Ensure compliance with regulatory guidelines for shelf life claims.

Packaging Tips for Commercial Use

• USE STERILE, AIRTIGHT, and labeled bottles with dispensers for easy and hygienic use.

• Clearly mention usage instructions and storage guidance on the packaging.

Unique Selling Proposition (USP)

• HIGHLIGHT THE ORGANIC and natural composition suitable for all skin types.

• Emphasize the gentle yet effective makeup removal without harsh chemicals.

Creating an organic aloe vera makeup remover provides a gentle way to cleanse the skin. For commercial production, ensure compliance with cosmetic regulations, focus on organic qualities, and prioritize product safety and quality for an appealing commercial product.

DIY Organic Tinted Moisturizer: Natural Glow for Everyday Radiance

Ingredients

- Organic Facial Moisturizer: Hydrates and nourishes the skin. *(Quantity: 2 tablespoons)*
- Organic Aloe Vera Gel: Soothes and moisturizes the skin. *(Quantity: 1 tablespoon)*
- Organic Jojoba Oil: Balances skin oils and provides hydration. *(Quantity: 1 teaspoon)*
- Non-Nano Zinc Oxide Powder (for sunscreen, optional): Provides sun protection. *(Quantity: 1/2 teaspoon)*
- Organic Mineral Foundation Powder: Adds tint and coverage. *(Quantity: Varies based on desired coverage)*

Tools Required

- MIXING BOWL
- Measuring spoons
- Clean container with a pump or airtight lid for storage

Method

Homemade Version

Step 1: Mixing the Ingredients

IN A MIXING BOWL, COMBINE the facial moisturizer, aloe vera gel, and jojoba oil.

Optionally, if sun protection is desired, add non-nano zinc oxide powder and mix well.

Gradually add the mineral foundation powder, adjusting the quantity to achieve the desired coverage and tint. Mix thoroughly until all ingredients are well incorporated.

Step 2: Storing the Tinted Moisturizer

TRANSFER THE PREPARED tinted moisturizer into a clean container with a pump or an airtight lid for easy and hygienic use.

Store it in a cool, dry place away from direct sunlight.

Additional Tips

● APPLY THE TINTED moisturizer evenly onto clean skin using fingertips or a makeup sponge for a natural, radiant finish.

● Adjust the amount of mineral foundation powder to match your skin tone.

Caution

● PERFORM A PATCH test before regular use to ensure no skin irritation occurs.

Commercial Version

FOR COMMERCIAL PRODUCTION, consider:

Adjustments for Commercial Version

● INGREDIENTS FOR Commercial Version:

● Natural Preservatives: Add suitable natural preservatives to prolong shelf life. *(Quantity as per manufacturer's recommendation)*

- Emollients and Skin Enhancers: Incorporate additional skin-loving ingredients for added benefits, like antioxidants or plant extracts.

Shelf Life

- HOMEMADE: APPROXIMATELY 1-2 months if stored in a cool, dark place.
- Commercial: With added natural preservatives, shelf life can extend to 6-12 months. Ensure compliance with regulatory guidelines for shelf life claims.

Packaging Tips for Commercial Use

- USE STERILE, AIRTIGHT, and labeled containers with pumps or easy-to-use dispensers for customer convenience.
- Clearly indicate usage instructions, skin tone suitability, and key ingredients on the packaging.

Unique Selling Proposition (USP)

- HIGHLIGHT THE ORGANIC and natural composition suitable for daily use, offering hydration, coverage, and sun protection.
- Emphasize the customizable tint options to match various skin tones for a natural and flawless look.

Creating an organic tinted moisturizer offers a blend of hydration, coverage, and natural glow. For commercial production, ensure compliance with cosmetic regulations, focus on organic qualities, and prioritize product safety and quality for an appealing commercial product.

DIY Organic Shea Butter Tinted Moisturizer: Nourishing Radiance for Glowing Skin

Ingredients

- Organic Shea Butter: Provides deep hydration and skin nourishment. *(Quantity: 2 tablespoons)*
- Organic Aloe Vera Gel: Soothes and moisturizes the skin. *(Quantity: 1 tablespoon)*
- Organic Jojoba Oil: Balances skin oils and offers hydration. *(Quantity: 1 teaspoon)*
- Non-Nano Zinc Oxide Powder (for sunscreen, optional): Provides sun protection. *(Quantity: 1/2 teaspoon)*
- Organic Mineral Foundation Powder: Adds tint and coverage. *(Quantity: Varies based on desired coverage)*

Tools Required

- MIXING BOWL
- Measuring spoons
- Clean container with a pump or airtight lid for storage

Method

Homemade Version

Step 1: Blending the Ingredients

IN A MIXING BOWL, COMBINE organic shea butter, aloe vera gel, and jojoba oil.

Optionally, if sun protection is desired, add non-nano zinc oxide powder and mix well.

Gradually add the mineral foundation powder, adjusting the quantity to achieve the desired coverage and tint. Mix thoroughly until all ingredients are well incorporated.

Step 2: Storing the Tinted Moisturizer

TRANSFER THE PREPARED tinted moisturizer into a clean container with a pump or an airtight lid for easy and hygienic use.

Store it in a cool, dry place away from direct sunlight.

Additional Tips

• APPLY THE TINTED moisturizer onto clean skin using fingertips or a makeup sponge for a natural, radiant finish.

• Experiment with the amount of mineral foundation powder to match your skin tone perfectly.

Caution

• PERFORM A PATCH test before regular use to ensure no skin irritation occurs.

Commercial Version

FOR COMMERCIAL PRODUCTION, consider:

Adjustments for Commercial Version

• INGREDIENTS FOR Commercial Version:

• Natural Preservatives: Incorporate suitable natural preservatives to extend shelf life. *(Quantity as per manufacturer's recommendation)*

- Skin-Enhancing Ingredients: Add antioxidants or botanical extracts for additional skincare benefits.

Shelf Life

- HOMEMADE: APPROXIMATELY 1-2 months if stored in a cool, dark place.
- Commercial: With added natural preservatives, shelf life can extend to 6-12 months. Ensure compliance with regulatory guidelines for shelf life claims.

Packaging Tips for Commercial Use

- USE STERILE, AIRTIGHT, and labeled containers with pumps or easy-to-use dispensers for customer convenience.
- Clearly indicate usage instructions, skin tone suitability, and key ingredients on the packaging.

Unique Selling Proposition (USP)

- EMPHASIZE THE NOURISHING properties of organic shea butter for deep skin hydration and natural radiance.
- Highlight the customizable tint options to match various skin tones for a healthy and glowing complexion.

Creating an organic shea butter tinted moisturizer offers deep nourishment and a radiant glow. For commercial production, focus on complying with cosmetic regulations, ensuring product safety, and highlighting the organic and skincare benefits for an appealing commercial product.

DIY Organic Glitter Gel: Sparkling Glam for Fun Makeup Looks

Ingredients

- Organic Aloe Vera Gel: Provides a base and soothes the skin. *(Quantity: 2 tablespoons)*
- Organic Vegetable Glycerin: Enhances adhesion and adds moisture. *(Quantity: 1 teaspoon)*
- Organic Glitter: Adds sparkle and shine. *(Quantity: Varies based on desired glitter intensity)*
- Organic Essential Oil (optional): Provides fragrance and additional skincare benefits. *(Quantity: A few drops)*

Tools Required

- MIXING BOWL
- Measuring spoons
- Clean container with airtight lid for storage

Method

Homemade Version

Step 1: Mixing the Ingredients

IN A MIXING BOWL, COMBINE organic aloe vera gel and vegetable glycerin. Mix thoroughly.

Gradually add organic glitter to the mixture, adjusting the quantity based on your desired level of sparkle. Mix well to evenly distribute the glitter.

Step 2: Adding Essential Oil (Optional)

IF DESIRED, ADD A FEW drops of organic essential oil to add fragrance and enhance the skincare properties.

Mix the essential oil into the glitter gel mixture.

Step 3: Storing the Glitter Gel

TRANSFER THE PREPARED glitter gel into a clean container with an airtight lid for easy and hygienic use.

Store it in a cool, dry place away from direct sunlight.

Additional Tips

● EXPERIMENT WITH different sizes and colors of organic glitter for various makeup looks.

● Apply the glitter gel using fingertips or a makeup brush for precise application.

● A patch test is recommended before using the glitter gel on sensitive skin areas to check for any adverse reactions.

Caution

● AVOID CONTACT WITH eyes and sensitive areas. In case of irritation, discontinue use and rinse thoroughly with water.

Commercial Version

FOR COMMERCIAL PRODUCTION, consider:

Adjustments for Commercial Version

● INGREDIENTS FOR Commercial Version:

- Cosmetic-Grade Preservatives: Incorporate suitable preservatives for extended shelf life. *(Quantity as per manufacturer's recommendation)*

- FDA-Approved Glitters: Ensure the use of safe and approved glitters for cosmetics.

Shelf Life

- HOMEMADE: APPROXIMATELY 2-3 weeks if stored in a cool, dry place.
- Commercial: With added preservatives, shelf life can extend to 6-12 months. Comply with regulatory guidelines for shelf life claims.

Packaging Tips for Commercial Use

- USE STERILE, AIRTIGHT, and labeled containers with a dispenser for customer convenience.
- Clearly state usage instructions, avoid eye contact, and list key ingredients on the packaging.

Unique Selling Proposition (USP)

- EMPHASIZE THE ORGANIC and skin-friendly nature of the glitter gel suitable for fun and safe makeup applications.
- Highlight the versatility of the product for various makeup looks, festivals, parties, and artistic expressions.

Creating an organic glitter gel adds sparkle to your makeup routine. For commercial production, focus on safety, compliance with cosmetic regulations, and highlighting the organic, skin-friendly nature for an appealing commercial product.

DIY Organic Mica Powder Body Shimmer: Natural Radiance for Glowing Skin

Ingredients

- Organic Aloe Vera Gel: Provides a base and soothes the skin. *(Quantity: 2 tablespoons)*
- Organic Vegetable Glycerin: Enhances adhesion and adds moisture. *(Quantity: 1 teaspoon)*
- Organic Mica Powder: Adds shimmer and glow. *(Quantity: Varies based on desired shimmer intensity)*
- Organic Essential Oil (optional): Provides fragrance and additional skincare benefits. *(Quantity: A few drops)*

Tools Required

- MIXING BOWL
  - Measuring spoons
  - Clean container with airtight lid for storage

Method

Homemade Version

Step 1: Mixing the Ingredients

IN A MIXING BOWL, COMBINE organic aloe vera gel and vegetable glycerin. Mix thoroughly.

Gradually add organic mica powder to the mixture, adjusting the quantity based on your desired shimmer intensity. Mix well to evenly distribute the mica powder.

Step 2: Adding Essential Oil (Optional)

IF DESIRED, ADD A FEW drops of organic essential oil to add fragrance and enhance the skincare properties.

Mix the essential oil into the shimmer gel mixture.

Step 3: Storing the Body Shimmer

TRANSFER THE PREPARED shimmer gel into a clean container with an airtight lid for easy and hygienic use.

Store it in a cool, dry place away from direct sunlight.

Additional Tips

• EXPERIMENT WITH different shades of organic mica powder to create personalized shimmer effects.

• Apply the body shimmer onto the skin using fingertips or a makeup brush for a radiant and glowing appearance.

Caution

• AVOID APPLYING THE shimmer gel to broken or irritated skin. Perform a patch test to check for any skin reactions.

Commercial Version

FOR COMMERCIAL PRODUCTION, consider:

Adjustments for Commercial Version

• INGREDIENTS FOR Commercial Version:

• Natural Preservatives: Include suitable preservatives for prolonged shelf life. *(Quantity as per manufacturer's recommendation)*

- FDA-Approved Mica Powders: Ensure the use of safe and approved mica powders for cosmetics.

Shelf Life

- HOMEMADE: APPROXIMATELY 2-3 weeks if stored in a cool, dry place.
- Commercial: With added preservatives, shelf life can extend to 6-12 months. Adhere to regulatory guidelines for shelf life claims.

Packaging Tips for Commercial Use

- USE STERILE, AIRTIGHT, and labeled containers with an applicator for customer convenience.
- Clearly state usage instructions, avoid eye contact, and list key ingredients on the packaging.

Unique Selling Proposition (USP)

- HIGHLIGHT THE ORGANIC and natural qualities of the shimmer gel, providing a radiant glow without harsh chemicals.
- Emphasize the versatility of the product, suitable for various occasions, festivals, and adding glamour to everyday looks.

Crafting an organic mica powder body shimmer enhances your skin's natural radiance. For commercial production, prioritize safety, compliance with cosmetic regulations, and emphasize the organic, skin-friendly aspects for an appealing commercial product.

DIY Organic Glitter Dust: Sparkling Magic for Creative Makeup

Ingredients

- Organic Cornstarch: Provides a base and smooth texture. *(Quantity: 1 tablespoon)*
- Organic Mica Powder: Adds shimmer and color. *(Quantity: 1 teaspoon)*
- Organic Glitter: Adds sparkle and shine. *(Quantity: Varies based on desired glitter intensity)*
- Organic Jojoba Oil: Enhances adhesion and provides moisture. *(Quantity: A few drops)*

Tools Required

- MIXING BOWL
- Measuring spoons
- Clean container with a sifter or airtight lid for storage

Method

Homemade Version

Step 1: Mixing the Ingredients

IN A MIXING BOWL, COMBINE organic cornstarch and organic mica powder. Mix thoroughly to create the base.

Gradually add organic glitter to the base mixture, adjusting the quantity based on your desired level of sparkle. Mix well to evenly distribute the glitter.

Add a few drops of organic jojoba oil to the mixture and blend until you achieve a slightly damp, but not wet, consistency.

Step 2: Storing the Glitter Dust

TRANSFER THE PREPARED glitter dust into a clean container with a sifter or an airtight lid for easy and controlled application.

Store it in a cool, dry place away from direct sunlight.

Additional Tips

● EXPERIMENT WITH different colors and sizes of organic glitter and mica powder to create custom shades and effects.

● Apply the glitter dust using a makeup brush or fingertips for a shimmering finish on eyes, cheeks, or body.

Caution

● AVOID USING GLITTER near the eyes or on sensitive areas. In case of irritation, discontinue use and wash off thoroughly with water.

Commercial Version

FOR COMMERCIAL PRODUCTION, consider:

Adjustments for Commercial Version

● INGREDIENTS FOR Commercial Version:

● Natural Preservatives: Incorporate suitable preservatives to extend shelf life. *(Quantity as per manufacturer's recommendation)*

● Cosmetic-Grade Glitters: Ensure the use of safe and approved glitters suitable for cosmetics.

Shelf Life

● HOMEMADE: APPROXIMATELY 2-3 months if stored in a cool, dry place.

● Commercial: With added preservatives, shelf life can extend to 6-12 months. Comply with regulatory guidelines for shelf life claims.

Packaging Tips for Commercial Use

● USE STERILE, LABELED containers with a sifter or an applicator for customer convenience.

● Clearly state usage instructions, avoid eye contact, and list key ingredients on the packaging.

Unique Selling Proposition (USP)

● EMPHASIZE THE ORGANIC and natural qualities of the glitter dust for safe and glamorous makeup applications.

● Highlight the versatility of the product suitable for artistic makeup, festivals, parties, and creative expressions.

Crafting an organic glitter dust adds sparkle to your makeup routine. For commercial production, focus on safety, compliance with cosmetic regulations, and highlight the organic, skin-friendly nature for an appealing commercial product.

DIY Organic Rosewater Face Mist: Refreshing Floral Elixir for Your Skin

Ingredients

- Organic Rose Petals: Provide natural fragrance and skin-soothing properties. *(Quantity: 1 cup)*
- Distilled Water: Serves as a solvent for extracting the essence of rose petals. *(Quantity: 2 cups)*
- Organic Vegetable Glycerin: Adds moisture and helps retain skin hydration. *(Quantity: 1 tablespoon)*
- Organic Witch Hazel: Acts as a natural astringent and toner. *(Quantity: 1 tablespoon)*
- Organic Essential Oil (optional): Enhances fragrance and provides additional skin benefits. *(Quantity: A few drops)*

Tools Required

- SAUCEPAN WITH LID
  - Heat-resistant bowl
  - Fine-mesh strainer
  - Clean spray bottle for storage

Method

Homemade Version

Step 1: Making Rosewater Infusion

IN A SAUCEPAN, COMBINE the organic rose petals and distilled water. Cover and simmer on low heat for about 20-30 minutes until the petals lose their color.

Remove the saucepan from heat and allow the mixture to cool completely.

Strain the rosewater infusion using a fine-mesh strainer into a heat-resistant bowl, discarding the used rose petals.

Step 2: Adding Additional Ingredients

ONCE THE ROSEWATER infusion has cooled, add organic vegetable glycerin and organic witch hazel. Stir well to combine.

If desired, add a few drops of organic essential oil for enhanced fragrance and additional skin benefits. Stir gently.

Step 3: Storing the Face Mist

TRANSFER THE PREPARED rosewater face mist into a clean spray bottle for easy and convenient use.

Store it in the refrigerator to prolong its shelf life and for a refreshing spritz.

Additional Tips

• USE THE ROSEWATER face mist as a hydrating toner, makeup setting spray, or a refreshing mist throughout the day for a boost of moisture and fragrance.

• Perform a patch test before applying the mist to your face to check for any adverse reactions.

Caution

• IF YOU HAVE SENSITIVE skin or are allergic to roses, consult with a dermatologist before using this face mist.

Commercial Version

FOR COMMERCIAL PRODUCTION, consider:

Adjustments for Commercial Version

● INGREDIENTS FOR Commercial Version:

   ● Natural Preservatives: Include suitable preservatives for prolonged shelf life. *(Quantity as per manufacturer's recommendation)*

Shelf Life

● HOMEMADE: APPROXIMATELY 1-2 weeks when stored in the refrigerator due to absence of preservatives.
   ● Commercial: With added preservatives, shelf life can extend to 6-12 months. Comply with regulatory guidelines for shelf life claims.

Packaging Tips for Commercial Use

● USE CLEAN, LABELED spray bottles with a fine mist nozzle for easy and controlled application.
   ● Highlight the organic and natural aspects of the product on the packaging to attract eco-conscious consumers.

Unique Selling Proposition (USP)

● EMPHASIZE THE ORGANIC and skin-friendly nature of the rosewater face mist, offering a refreshing and hydrating solution with natural floral fragrance.

Creating an organic rosewater face mist provides a rejuvenating experience for your skin. For commercial production, focus on safety, compliance with cosmetic regulations, and emphasize the organic, skin-friendly aspects for an appealing commercial product.

DIY Organic Green Tea Face Mist: Revitalize Your Skin with Nature's Goodness

Ingredients

- Organic Green Tea Leaves: Rich in antioxidants, rejuvenates the skin. *(Quantity: 2 tablespoons)*
- Distilled Water: Acts as a solvent to extract the benefits of green tea. *(Quantity: 1 cup)*
- Organic Aloe Vera Gel: Soothes and hydrates the skin. *(Quantity: 2 tablespoons)*
- Organic Essential Oil (optional): Adds fragrance and extra skincare benefits. *(Quantity: A few drops)*

Tools Required

- SAUCEPAN WITH LID
  - Heat-resistant bowl
  - Fine-mesh strainer
  - Clean spray bottle for storage

Method

Homemade Version

Step 1: Brewing Green Tea Infusion

IN A SAUCEPAN, BRING distilled water to a gentle boil. Remove from heat.

Add organic green tea leaves to the hot water and cover the saucepan. Steep for about 10-15 minutes to extract the goodness of green tea.

Strain the green tea infusion using a fine-mesh strainer into a heat-resistant bowl, allowing it to cool completely.

Step 2: Adding Additional Ingredients

ONCE THE GREEN TEA infusion has cooled, add organic aloe vera gel to the bowl. Mix well to combine.

Optionally, add a few drops of organic essential oil for added fragrance and skincare benefits. Stir gently.

Step 3: Storing the Face Mist

TRANSFER THE PREPARED green tea face mist into a clean spray bottle for easy application.

Store it in the refrigerator for a refreshing and soothing mist.

Additional Tips

● USE THE GREEN TEA face mist as a toner after cleansing or throughout the day to refresh and revitalize your skin.

● Conduct a patch test before applying it to your face to ensure compatibility with your skin.

Caution

● AVOID USING THE face mist if you have any allergies to green tea or any other ingredients. Discontinue use if irritation occurs.

Commercial Version

FOR COMMERCIAL PRODUCTION, consider:

Adjustments for Commercial Version

● INGREDIENTS FOR Commercial Version:

● Natural Preservatives: Include suitable preservatives for longer shelf life. *(Quantity as per manufacturer's recommendation)*

Shelf Life

- HOMEMADE: APPROXIMATELY 1-2 weeks when stored in the refrigerator due to absence of preservatives.
- Commercial: With added preservatives, shelf life can extend to 6-12 months. Adhere to regulatory guidelines for shelf life claims.

Packaging Tips for Commercial Use

- USE CLEAN, LABELED spray bottles with a fine mist nozzle for easy application.
- Emphasize the organic and natural properties on the packaging to appeal to eco-conscious consumers.

Unique Selling Proposition (USP)

- HIGHLIGHT THE ANTIOXIDANT-rich organic green tea and soothing organic aloe vera in the mist for a natural and refreshing skincare experience.

Crafting an organic green tea face mist provides a refreshing boost for your skin. For commercial production, focus on safety, compliance with cosmetic regulations, and highlight the organic, skin-loving qualities for an attractive commercial product.

DIY Organic Lavender Face Mist: Nourish Your Skin with Nature's Serenity

Ingredients

- Organic Lavender Flowers: Renowned for soothing properties and a calming aroma. *(Quantity: 2 tablespoons)*
- Distilled Water: Serves as a solvent to infuse lavender's benefits. *(Quantity: 1 cup)*
- Organic Witch Hazel: A natural astringent that balances and tones the skin. *(Quantity: 2 tablespoons)*
- Organic Vegetable Glycerin: Offers hydration and retains moisture. *(Quantity: 1 tablespoon)*
- Organic Lavender Essential Oil: Enhances fragrance and adds to the calming effect. *(Quantity: A few drops)*

Tools Required

- SAUCEPAN WITH LID
- Heat-resistant bowl
- Fine-mesh strainer
- Clean spray bottle for storage

Method

Homemade Version

Step 1: Infusing Lavender

HEAT DISTILLED WATER in a saucepan until it's warm but not boiling.

Add organic lavender flowers to the warm water, cover the saucepan, and let it steep for about 10-15 minutes.

Strain the lavender-infused water using a fine-mesh strainer into a heat-resistant bowl. Allow it to cool completely.

Step 2: Adding Skincare Ingredients

ONCE COOLED, ADD ORGANIC witch hazel to the lavender-infused water in the bowl. Mix well.

Incorporate organic vegetable glycerin into the mixture, stirring gently.

Add a few drops of organic lavender essential oil for a heightened fragrance and extra calming effect. Stir to combine evenly.

Step 3: Storing the Face Mist

TRANSFER THE PREPARED lavender face mist into a clean spray bottle for convenient use.

Store it in a cool, dark place, away from direct sunlight.

Additional Tips

- USE THE LAVENDER face mist as a refreshing toner or as a relaxing spritz to calm your skin and senses.
- Perform a patch test before applying it generously to your face to ensure compatibility with your skin.

Caution

- DISCONTINUE USE if any irritation or adverse reactions occur.
- Avoid use if you have known allergies to lavender or any ingredients in the recipe.

Commercial Version

FOR COMMERCIAL PRODUCTION:

Adjustments for Commercial Version

- INGREDIENTS FOR Commercial Version:

• Natural Preservatives: Include appropriate preservatives to extend shelf life. *(Quantity as per industry standards)*

Shelf Life

• HOMEMADE: APPROXIMATELY 1-2 weeks when stored in a cool place due to the absence of preservatives.
• Commercial: With added preservatives, shelf life can extend to 6-12 months. Follow regulatory guidelines for shelf life claims.

Packaging Tips for Commercial Use

• USE STERILE, LABELED spray bottles to ensure hygiene and easy application.
• Highlight the organic and calming properties on the packaging to appeal to consumers seeking natural skincare products.

Unique Selling Proposition (USP)

• EMPHASIZE THE ORGANIC lavender's calming and soothing benefits, promoting relaxation and skin nourishment.

Creating an organic lavender face mist provides a rejuvenating and serene skincare experience. For commercial production, focus on safety, regulatory compliance, and highlight the natural, calming qualities for an appealing product.